FIT
ACTIVE & AGELESS FOR LIFE

KELLY HOWARD

FIT
Active & Ageless for Life
Copyright @ 2023. Kelly Howard, Events Cafe LLC. All rights reserved. No part of this book may be reproduced by any mechanical, photographic, or electronic process or in the form of a phonographic recording; nor may it be stored in a retrieval system, transmitted, or otherwise be copied for public or private use—other than for "fair use" as brief quotations embodied in articles and reviews—without prior written permission of the publisher.

This publication is designed to provide accurate and authoritative information regarding the subject matter covered. It is sold with the understanding that the publisher is not engaged in rendering legal, accounting, or other professional services. If you require legal advice or other expert assistance, you should seek the services of a competent professional.

Design and cover art by Oladimeja
Editor: Fatima Alishba

Disclaimer: The author makes no guarantees to the results you'll achieve by reading this book. All fitness requires risk and hard work. The results and client case studies presented in this book represent results achieved working directly with the author. Your results may vary when undertaking any new fitness or health strategy.

To the women in Fit is Freedom.

You inspire, delight, and never fail to amaze me. No matter the path each of you hikes, you are always moving toward your North Star and inspiring those around you. I love each and every one of you.

Hugs - Kelly

"Fitness is a long game. It's not something you do until you hit a goal, like losing weight. It's a way of living for the rest of your life. The reason so many diets fail and workouts don't work is we over-plan and under-act. We believe that fitness is a goal when in fact, it's a journey." Kelly

Contents

Introduction 8

PART 1

CHAPTER 1
The View from the Mountain Top 16

CHAPTER 2
This Book Is For You If… 22

Exercise #1: The Starting Line 30

CHAPTER 3
The Five Consistency Killers 35

Exercise #2: Recognizing and Avoiding Consistency Killers 45

CHAPTER 4
Your North Star 50

Exercise #3: Living life in full color 57

CHAPTER 5
Fitness - There Are No Shortcuts 60

Exercise #4: Eliminating the Quick Fixes 68

PART 2

CHAPTER 6
A Life of Freedom Begins by Design 72

Exercise #5: Set Yourself Up to Win 77

CHAPTER 7
Creating Your Custom Fitness Plan 81

CHAPTER 7.5
Starting and Staying Consistent 117

CHAPTER 8
Forget Changing Habits: Simply Shift Them! 127

PART 3

CHAPTER 9
Smashing Excuses 142

CHAPTER 10
Accountability: The Good, the Bad, and the Stop it Right Now! 154

CHAPTER 11
The Toolbox 164

CHAPTER 12
The Four Fitness Pillars 181

CHAPTER 13
Sometimes It Might Hurt 189

CHAPTER 14
Your Road Map to Fitness Freedom 198

Book Bonuses 202

About Kelly 205

FREE DOWNLOAD

Before you dive in, please download your editable Freedom Journal. As you go through the book, you'll find that it simplifies tracking your notes, ideas, and fitness plan as you follow along.

FitisFreedom.com/Bonuses

As a reader, you will also find several helpful videos and downloads to make your fitness path even easier.

INTRODUCTION

> *"Welcome, I'm so glad you're here. Since you've picked up this book, I know you've made the decision to focus on your fitness and health. Kudos. As you read through this book, years of unspoken rules that led you to put your desires on the backburner will begin to fade, and you'll feel a profound shift. Forget ever giving up or throwing in the towel. It's your time to shine, and I'm so glad we're on this journey together. Never accept less than what you truly desire. Hugs"* — Kelly

You awake just a few short weeks after you have read and applied this book. Feeling amazing, you notice your energy is high, and you're ready for the new day. Smiling, you think about the upcoming adventures you have planned, adventures that at one time were only a dream.

Life is good.

And, when you feel good, it's easy to do great things. Everyone's "great things" are different. For you, it could be traveling to all the places you've always wanted to go. Or, it could be playing with the grandkids and meeting whatever challenge they throw your way with a big smile. Or, it could be participating in active adventures like hiking, kayaking, and cycling. Or, maybe, you want to pass a mirror and smile at the image you see.

Everything you want is possible.

In this book, you'll hear about the good, bad, and ugly of my own journey and what many of my clients have experienced. Just like my clients, I have your absolute best interest at heart. I'll cheer you on and, with a bit of tough love, call you out on your excuses if needed.

You'll find the more you follow my **Fit is Freedom Formula** outlined within this book, the more possibilities and hope life will deliver.

I'm here to help you in two ways.

1. To help you become healthy, fit, and vibrant so you can achieve and live the adventurous life you crave, no matter your starting point today.
2. To equip you with everything I've learned over the last twenty-plus years that will help you stay consistent with your fitness. If you never again catch yourself saying, "I'll start next week," I've done my job!

In order to make you fitness consistent, I've structured this book as follows:

First, let's get an honest picture of where you are today. When you understand precisely where you're starting from and what you bring to the process, it will be much easier to follow my specific guidance and advice. Throughout the book, you'll complete many self-assessments to help you know the best ways to proceed. These assessments are quick and based on my 20-plus years of working with women, helping them reach their fitness and adventure goals through coaching, training, and cheering them on. Please don't skip them. In fact, you'll find an editable Freedom Journal that will help you follow along with ease at www.FitisFreedom.com/Bonuses

Next, I'll share how creating a plan specifically tailored to your life and body will change everything you have thought about fitness. At each stage in life, we need the right plan for who we are at that moment, not a cookie-cutter suggestion from some Instagram Goddess' post!

We'll look at the role our thoughts play in our fitness. We'll uncover why you move forward in leaps and bounds when you have your mind on board with your fitness and health goals. You'll also learn why no one addresses the importance of engaging your brain in getting the body you desire.

Along with the good stuff, we'll take a look at what's been holding you back and why you might *not really* want to focus on your fitness. We'll uncover where you are wasting time on an emotional roller coaster of hope, action, inaction, and disappointment. And, more importantly, how to exit that roller coaster ride for good!

Next, I'll share with you steps and strategies from the **Fit is Freedom Formula.** This is the method I personally use to help my clients succeed in creating fitness consistency that sticks with ease, no matter what problems or roadblocks life throws your way. I love sharing these steps and seeing the magic they create.

We will build the foundation you need and learn how to upgrade your fitness plan when the time is right. Plus, you'll learn how to develop the motivation, accountability, and community that is the bedrock of **the Fit is Freedom Formula**. I'll show you how to put your plan together in an easy, step-by-step process you can uplevel as your fitness grows.

My goal is for you to have a plan and to take action long before you finish reading this book!

Finally, we'll come full circle, and I'll show you how to stay on track and reignite your fitness goals again and again, no matter what life throws your way.

What to Expect by the End of this Book:
1: You'll have a North Star.

When you have a goal that resonates deep in your soul, that goal is emotionally charged and easier to strive for. You'll learn why most fitness goals fall flat, and you'll develop new goals with heart. Goals that shine and give you a guiding light to reach for. You will drop the "shoulds" or "need to" and focus on what matters the most for you. In finding your star, you'll find the fit future You.

2: A custom plan designed for you, by you.

You'll understand why cookie-cutter fitness plans don't work. Injuries, boredom, and lack of results happen when you follow something designed for **anybody** instead of designed for **your body**. When you follow the Fit is Freedom Formula, you'll have a simple, fun plan custom designed to change as your body changes.

3: You will learn to prioritize fitness.

As busy, successful women, we've spent most of our life helping and caring for others. At first, prioritizing our fitness can feel a little selfish or uncaring for everyone who needs us and our time. You'll come to find that prioritizing your fitness is the most unselfish and loving action you can give to yourself and the ones you love.

4: You will have all the tools you need to stop you from ever straying off course again.

Motivation is a learned behavior, and habits can shift. As you apply all the tools you learn throughout this book, you'll be prepared for the roadblocks and circumstances life brings your way!

The method you're about to discover has radically transformed my life and the lives of thousands of my clients, with benefits radically beyond losing weight, fitting into last decade's jeans, dumping the menopause middle, or getting your energy back.

I sincerely believe that when we prioritize our fitness and health, we "put our oxygen mask on first," and the ripple effect is astronomical. We live longer, healthier lives and can be there 100% for the people in our lives. We're role models for the people we love, especially the young ones. We no longer focus on what might go wrong because we are too busy living lives that are going right! Over the years, I've found that the women I attract are a lot like me, and freedom is a driver. This book will help you create that freedom.

Because…being **Fit is Freedom.** It is time to turn back the clock. To start living a life brimming with possibilities. To have more to look forward to than you ever thought possible. We're living in exciting times. The science and cutting-edge knowledge of how to live vibrantly into our 70's, 80's, 90's, and beyond is here. The understanding that fitness, strength, flexibility, and mental acuity contribute to our lifespan is common knowledge. And yet, learning to apply everything we know easily and consistently isn't common knowledge. This is where I come in.

Helping amazing women like you create lives filled with fitness, fun, and freedom is what I do best. As you read this book, if you find yourself ready to create the life you desire and require my personal help, I'm here for you. You can book a chat by going to:

FitisFreedom.com/call

Thank you so much for joining me and all the women in the Fit is Freedom community. I'm so excited to be on this journey together. ~ Kelly

DISCLAIMER AKA COMMON SENSE NOTES

Before starting this or any other fitness program, consult your physician or other health care professional to determine if it is appropriate for your specific needs. This is particularly important if you (or your family) have a history of high blood pressure or heart disease, or if you have ever experienced chest pain when exercising or have experienced chest pain in the past month when not engaged in physical activity, smoke, have high cholesterol, are obese, or have a bone or joint problem that could be worsened by physical activity.

If your physician or healthcare provider advises against starting this fitness program, you should not begin it. Additionally, if you experience any symptoms such as faintness, dizziness, pain, or shortness of breath while exercising, you should stop immediately.

This book is intended for educational purposes only and provides health and fitness information. The information presented should not be relied upon as a substitute for, nor does it replace, professional medical advice, diagnosis, or treatment.

Always consult with a physician or other healthcare professional regarding any concerns or questions about your health. Do not disregard, avoid, or delay obtaining medical or health-related advice from your healthcare professional because of something you may have read in this book. The use of any information provided in this book is at your own risk, and you should not use it as a substitute for professional advice. Do not act upon or rely on this information without seeking professional advice first.

Please note that individual circumstances vary, and the information in this book is the author's personal opinion. Transmission of this information is not intended to create a professional-client relationship between Fit is Freedom/ Events Cafe LLC and you. The owners, editors, contributors, administrators, and other staff of Events Cafe LLC are not qualified professionals, and the information contained in this book should not be construed as professional advice.

PART 1

CHAPTER 1
THE VIEW FROM THE MOUNTAIN TOP

The view was breathtaking as we stood shoulder to shoulder at the top of the trail, looking out over the spectacular vista. We were sweaty, breathless, red-faced, and smiling from ear to ear. The hike had been harder than I had planned, but everyone aced it. As we stood together, taking in the sights, joking, teasing each other, and making outrageous plans for everything we would eat for dinner, my mind jumped back to four short months earlier, the moment this trip had been born.

For several months I had been thinking about inviting the women in the Fit is Freedom group on a hiking retreat in my favorite place in the States; the green, lush, fog-filled Smoky Mountains of the Southeast. I had even picked a date and found a luxurious private home to rent, but I wasn't sure if this was something the crew would enjoy doing? I knew it was something most of the women had never done before. It would certainly be a stretch physically and mentally, but as I am fond of saying, *if you're not pushing yourself, you're slipping backward.* While we were on a group coaching call wrapping up a month of Sugar Freedom, everyone was high on the accomplishment of no sugar for a month, and they wanted to know, "What was next?"

So I tossed out…"Who wants to join me on a hiking trip in the Smoky Mountains?"

After a resounding unanimous YES, I gave them the dates and showed them the house I had found; everyone was in. I booked our private home while on the call, and the retreat was on!

Done and done.

As I looked around our Zoom gallery, I could see anxious thoughts beginning to cross people's minds and faces, and I could only guess what they were thinking…

"What the hell did I just agree to do?"

"What if I can't keep up?"

"What if I hold everyone back?"

"Oh my, I have never done something like this before; what was I thinking?!?"

Over the next four months, everyone diligently followed our online training plan as we trained for the trails virtually and held each other accountable in the group. We cheered each other on, felt each other's pain, and our excitement grew for what was to come. As we descended upon the Smokies, everyone already had stories to share before a single step was taken!

I have changed all the names for the sake of privacy, but let me share their wonderful stories.

J said her grown kids were worried sick about this trip. What was she thinking? Were we safe to be with? Was she going to be safe? She didn't even know us; personally, she'd never been on a hiking or adventure trip before, and what if she got lost or couldn't keep up?

(spoiler alert - she did amazing, blazing the trails and fitting in like a long-lost sister)

H had been an athlete all her life but had struggled with injuries for the past several years and wasn't sure her body would hold up for the entire trip. She did awesome, of course, and pitched in to help everyone else along the way.

S was afraid she would be too slow, that despite the training, she just wasn't a fast hiker. So what? She had a ball! She took brilliant photos and made sure everyone followed the right trails and stopped to admire the beauty along the way. It was a perfect first hiking trip.

F had a great fitness foundation, but due to her hectic work schedule, she hadn't put in the training time she hoped to get done. It didn't matter as she romped along the trails. As I often say, once you have a true fitness foundation, you never need to worry. Our bodies are amazingly resilient, and we're made to play!

L had packed on extra weight over the last couple of years, which was weighing her down and impeding her progress. As she trained for the trip, she found weight coming off, but even better, she began to feel stronger and fitter than she had in years. The crazy thing was that we only trained for four months, yet it was like two years of stress and aging simply fell away for her!

Now, your path may not be to hike the Smokies (but we go every year, and I can't wait to invite you if this is a dream trip for you). You may find that you have other desires.

You might be like Amy, who joined Fit is Freedom because she wanted to be a part of her grandchildren's lives for a very, very long time, but she was beginning to have trouble keeping up with them. She wanted to be the grandmother who did all the fun trips and activities, but she needed to get back in shape. Amy started very small, with consistent walks and just a little mobility because she hadn't done much of anything in years. As she became more confident, we focused on her strength and capacity, and within just a few short months, she was in the pool tossing those grandkids around!

Or maybe, like Julie, you have had a myriad of joint issues, body aches, pain, or even surgeries. You're not ready to buy the "it's time to slow down" story. You are ready to do what you must to live a fit and pain-free life for a very long time.

Or maybe you're like Paula, a busy CEO who runs a company that was running her into the ground. She was waking up tired, out of energy at the end of the day, and compensating with caffeine and sugar that wreaked havoc on her sleep and stomach. She was frazzled and exhausted and knew she had to stop wearing her body down, but she didn't know where to start or how to get back on track. After learning how to manage her sugar cravings and adding the right cardio to her lifestyle, she has turned her life around. Now she wakes up feeling refreshed after a great night's sleep, the constant headaches have disappeared, and she's more successful in her business than ever. She no longer feels guilty focusing on her fitness first because she sees that her new lifestyle leads to even greater success.

Or, maybe you're like Sue, who came to me when she had reached a breaking point. She was ready to give up trying, to throw in the towel because the vibrant, healthy life she dreamed of felt so far away it was lost to her.

We all have our own story. Tell me, what is your path, and where do you want to go?

Fit is Free Friend – Susie

"Fitness [to me] used to mean...how do I look in my clothes 😊 and now it means being strong enough to do things I want to do. Being in better condition so I don't get hurt when I'm doing the things I love to do.

Having flexibility, strength, and stamina, so I can do fun, active outdoor activities and eat what I want to eat!" - Susie

Susie wanted to be the "Cool Grandma." The one all the kids came to for fun, adventures, and exciting stuff. But deep down, she wanted more than that. She wanted to look great, have more fun and adventure, and live the life she had always dreamed of, but joint pain, lack of sleep, and poor food and drink choices stood in her way.

When we first started working together, fitness was all about being slender and fitting into her clothes. And she told me she would probably need shoulder surgery soon; her shoulder bothered her all the time, oh and by the way, she wasn't doing any weights. They just bored her. :) She liked to walk, and that was it.

So I smiled and asked her, *"How's that working for you?"*

We had a good laugh because we both knew that just walking with no mobility, no adjustments to her food as fuel (we'll talk more about this in later chapters), and with sarcopenia (muscle loss from age) looming, **something had to change**. It was time for a line in the sand. Get strong to live long, or start fading away.

She chose **change**.

Together, we created a plan that she approved of! In the past, she'd tried working with fitness trainers, but they were too regimented for her, and she needed options. We focused on walking, resistance with bands, and yoga. And we started small with the bands because she was worried about her shoulder and hadn't worked out with any resistance in decades.

As Susie began to get stronger, joints that had bothered her for years ached less, and even more interestingly, her shoulder hurt less and less.

(Note: Your plan has to be something you like, or you won't do it. If it's not fun, it's not sustainable. This doesn't mean everything in your fitness plan needs to feel like a party, but you have to enjoy most of it.)

After working together for a few months, it was time for a more significant challenge, so I asked her - *"if you could do anything, if you were fit enough to do something that sounds amazing to you, what would you do"?*

Bam, no hesitation.

"I'd be one of those women who aren't afraid to go traveling, even alone. Someone who walks on a plane with her head held high because she's confident and strong. She tosses her backpack in the overhead bin without a thought because, well, because she is strong and doesn't need anyone's help."

Fast forward five months, and we're hiking the Appalachian trail, side by side, with Susie surging ahead at times. She's hit her stride, and nothing is slowing her down.

In case you're wondering…when she got on the plane to join me in the Smokies, she tossed that heavy pack into the overhead bin like it was nothing while wearing a big, I-can-do-anything grin!

If you're "Oh my gosh, I need to learn more right this minute," :) Find a spot on my calendar, and let's see how I can help: FitisFreedom.com/call

CHAPTER 2
THIS BOOK IS FOR YOU IF...

My calling as a fitness consistency expert began in an unconventional and very uncomfortable way; flat on my back, doubled up in discomfort, and unable to move.

My journey started the day I woke up in too much pain to get out of bed.

Unable to walk because of the pain, I literally crawled on my hands and knees to the bathroom and then back into bed, where I stayed for several days. I spent hours online researching anything that could fit the bill - slipped disc, kidney stones, you name it, I googled it. In a crazy half-kidding but not really kidding kind of way, I was almost desperate to find something seriously wrong. Some kind of illness where I could just go to the doctor and say, "Here, you fix this!"

Because the truth was, intuitively, I already knew what was wrong. And it absolutely terrified me.

Simply put, I had put my health on the back burner and was trying to get by instead of living a life filled with health and thriving.

I had made everyone and everything else my priority. My health was in the toilet because I'd fallen for the "next week" myth. Next week was when I'd get my act together and my time back; that's when I'd start focusing on my fitness again.

That was a BS decision for someone who had been an athlete most of her adult life!

Fueled on nothing but coffee and takeout meals, I was spending 12-14 hour days hunched over my laptop, precariously perched on a piece of plywood in the middle of an unbuilt kitchen, as I juggled my growing business while acting as the general contractor on our new home remodeling, and at the same time caring for my mom who was now in a wheelchair and needed extra support. I was wearing all of the hats, doing all of the things for everyone else. I was absolutely stressed out of my mind.

Want to know the real kicker? The company I was so invested in building - it was an outdoor adventure company. Not only were my weekends spent leading 40-mile bike rides, daylong hikes, and kayaking trips, I was supposed to be the model for healthy, outdoor adventuring!

I had become a "do as I say, not as I do" person as I assured everyone that being a weekend warrior was not a good practice. They needed to be moving during the week, not just on the weekends.

(Some things are hard to admit)

My behavior was completely unsustainable, and I absolutely knew it. But like so many busy women, I pushed through – promising myself that if I could just get through this season of craziness, then everything would settle down, and I could start to focus on myself and my fitness again.

But that moment of calm never came, and amid everything that was going on, it was only a matter of time until my body revolted – and so when it finally did, in a rather spectacular fashion, it became apparent that it was time to make lasting changes.

As I lay in bed, popping Advil to fight off the pain, I couldn't help but reflect on how I ended up in this state. I used to be so active, and this body, which currently felt immobilized, was once my vehicle for incredible adventures. I had conquered the Athens to Atlanta 86-mile skate race, completed grueling 100-mile bike rides in a single day, and even tackled mountain bike races. I even tried my hand at Whitewater kayaking with some success, while surfing remains an ongoing (and, so far, unsuccessful) endeavor. Each of these adventures taught me valuable lessons on training and recovery, on maintaining a flexible, vibrant, and energized body.

So what happened? And, more importantly, how could I get back to being that person who prioritized her health? The one who focused on her fitness consistency, who scheduled her workouts and treated food as fuel, not comfort.

The more I thought about it, the more I realized that almost every woman I knew was in a similar position to me. Too busy taking care of everyone and everything else that there was simply no time left to take care of themselves. Pushing off their own needs with the best intention of getting around to it next week, next month, and even sadly next year, the years piled on, and fitness was fading.

Everyone was waiting for something external in their life to change before they could make the changes they needed to make.

The job needed to change so they could work less

The kids needed to go back to school (or get out of school)

They needed to recover from an injury or have surgery

They needed to lose weight so they'd have the energy to work out

They needed to quit caring for their mother, in-laws, insert your person here…

At that moment, I decided that I was done waiting and ready to completely change my life and the way I was living. Vowing to get back to my roots and everything I knew about getting and staying healthy, it was "line in the sand" time.

And that's precisely what happened. As I focused on my wellness and fitness, slowly and surely, my life began to turn around. Fast-forward several years, and I can now say that 90% of the time, I do exactly what I need to do to stay on track with my fitness. And 90% is the key because, as you'll learn later, 100% absolute perfection will derail your fitness goals every single time.

I knew my situation wasn't unique, and I wanted to take my story and success to other women. So began my real journey as a fitness consistency coach. My friends became my willing guinea pigs. Everyone was desperately trying to figure out how to make the changes they needed and fiercely create the results they wanted. They were so over losing the same fifteen pounds or waking up tired and then going to bed still tired. Quite frankly, we're all at an age where it is time to quit messing around and start creating lasting change. There is no time to take actions that never work.

What began as a small accountability group of five has grown into a movement of thousands of women who embrace the Fit is Freedom Formula. Women who are enjoying lives filled with fun, fitness, and freedom. Women who are looking forward to everything that feeling great and being fit gives them.

The most powerful step you can take today to change your future is to learn how to get off of the stop-start-stop-start-again rollercoaster that fitness and, thus, health have become for so many women. We were taught to put everyone and everything else first, and now it's time for your own "line in the sand moment."

Are you ready to completely change the trajectory of your future?

The awesome-crazy thing is you don't have to spend hours lifting weights at a gym (unless that's your jam), start running marathons (or even 5k's), or never enjoy a donut again, although you may choose not to, and that's your decision!

You don't have to spend hours on your fitness, but you will need to learn to become strategic about what you do. I'll help you create your specific plan in Part 2. In the meantime, just know that you'll learn to use a mixture of cardio, resistance, and mobility, and the options to choose from are unlimited!

You'll learn how to create an MDM (Minimum Daily Movement) that fits your lifestyle and a Maximum. Yes, there is a point where too much movement actually works against us. At a certain point, typically around midlife or menopause, our body composition begins to change, and what used to work for weight loss no longer does.

You will counterbalance these changes by learning how to use what I like to call a **cascading effect of good.** Every good action you add to your plan will lead to an exponentially better outcome.

Add into your routine a mobility that you love and your joints will hurt less, your stress levels will reduce, and your cortisol belly fat will start disappearing. Your sleep will also improve, which is one of the most important things you can do to stay healthy. I'm all for sleeping our way to health. ☺

When you add in the right resistance training, your body composition will improve, your metabolism will increase, your bones will strengthen, and your balance will improve. A double dose of a cascading effect of good as you naturally reverse aging!

As joints hurt less and the extra weight disappears, the joy of cardio really kicks in. Whatever you have dreamed of doing, hiking, kayaking, standup paddling boarding, or throwing the kids around in the pool, any and all of the wonderful adventures to be had become easier to do. And you'll be inspired to do them.

When you become consistent with your fitness. When you no longer have a hit-or-miss relationship with your health, you'll feel better, look better, and naturally have more fun.

I promise.

Our bodies are resilient, and it's time to give your body what it needs to flourish.

This Book is For You If...

This book is for you if you're tired of saying you'll start next week, next month, when the current project is over, or when the stars align!

- This book is for you if you start a workout plan only to realize two weeks later you've already forgotten about what you started.

- This book is for you if you put everyone and everything else first, hoping that someday it will change and you'll find the time you desperately need for yourself.

- This book is for you if you wake up in the morning and it hurts – your back, neck, joints, knees, whatever, and you're secretly terrified that this is how you'll feel from here on out.

- This book is for you if you've tried everything before and nothing seems to stick. If you find yourself at square one, again and again, a little heavier, a little less energetic, and a lot more scared.

- This book is for you if you're gaining weight and losing muscle, and nothing you do seems to change this.

- This book is especially for you if you privately worry that this is as good as it will get, that maybe it really is time to throw in the towel.

Absolutely not.

I'm here to say that with a few changes, new tactics and know-how, having a plan designed for you, implementing simple habit shifts, the right accountability, and the right community, you'll be seeing big changes in no time at all.

You'll learn consistency tactics that work for you exactly where you are today. Easy methods to stay motivated, dedicated, and accountable even when you aren't feeling it. Plus, you'll uncover the secret sauce to having things to look forward to and connecting with the right community.

And the best part? This time it will stick because you have all the tools you need to create the life you desire. It's up to us to prioritize our health. Our bodies are amazingly resilient, and you will find that it doesn't take much, but it does take the right plan and the willingness to start with small, consistent steps.

I want your fitness to be simple. Simple is easy.

You'll learn to take the right actions, trust yourself, and approach your fitness differently than you ever had before.

The best part? We're going to make this fun. Because when it's fun, it's sustainable!

My Wish For You

I wish that in just a few short months, you'll wake one morning, stretching your arms over your head after a good night's sleep, feeling energized as your mind drifts back to the beginning of this journey. You whisper to yourself, "Wow, I feel amazing."

PART 1

As you bound out of bed, you know that by prioritizing your fitness and learning to stick to a movement plan based on your life and your body, you have shifted everything for yourself in a remarkable way! Your healthy lifestyle has become a habit, and you feel better than you have in years. Maybe even better than ever before. You have so much to look forward to and are excited about all the possibilities.

Welcome to the world of fitness consistency! A consistent woman is an action-taker, and it's your time to take a little action. Please grab your Freedom Journal (get your copy at www.FitisFreedom.com/bonuses and keep it with you on this entire journey). Do the quick Starting Line exercise in the next section. This will help you evaluate your current situation and determine your starting point. It will also help you build the right fitness foundation for yourself.

EXERCISE #1: THE STARTING LINE

It is so easy to discount what we have accomplished unless we track what we do. We think we'll remember, but we don't! Your accomplishments become a lot more apparent when you track things from the beginning and know your starting line.

Scales are capricious, and I believe there are better ways of scoring your fitness, like how you feel and what you can do! So take a few minutes and see where you are… In the exercise below, rate yourself on a scale of 1-5, 1 being "not accurate at all" and 5 being "most accurate." Total your score and use the answer key to determine your next steps.

What's Your Starting Line?

- I know exactly what I need to do to get in shape.
- I prioritize myself and my fitness.
- I schedule my workouts each week.
- I belong to a gym or have a space at my home for exercise.
- I smile when I pass a mirror and see myself.
- My closet is filled with clothes that fit.
- I like the way my clothes fit.
- When I think about my health, I feel great.
- I have almost zero aches or pains.
- I wake up refreshed and energetic.

What your score means:

- **Score 10 - 25**

    We met at the perfect time! Right now, you are putting the needs of everyone and everything before yourself, and you're either in burnout or heading there. Do not worry! We connected at the right time, and I love telling my clients and friends, "Our bodies are resilient." AND it's time to make time for yourself, your fitness, and your health. No different than the instructions on an airplane, put your oxygen mask on first before you take care of anyone else. When we take care of ourselves, we have more to give to those we love. Thank you for being here!

- **Score 26 - 40**

    It's your time to shine. Does it feel like you get started only to find yourself slipping backward, possibly again and again? But the best thing is that you keep trying, or at the minimum, you keep hoping. Having hope, seeing the possibilities in life, and taking small, clear steps is the perfect path to everything you want in life. One step in front of the other and keep reading, this book was written for you.

- **Score 41 - 50**

    Focusing on your fitness more lately? It's showing! The knowledge, know-how, and habit shifts in this book will serve to help you find more clarity on your journey. In the meantime, keep doing what you're doing, and let's take it up a notch; there is always more fun and fitness to be found in this one beautiful life we have.

Now that you know where you're starting from, let's look at what might hold you back. If fitness consistency were simply making a plan and then following through, we'd all have done it! Unfortunately, consistency is a struggle for most. We believe we struggle because we don't try hard enough. Nothing could be further from the truth! I know you've tried hard, and you've had some success. But, when success is short-lived, we must look at the real culprits, the actual consistency killers. Once you learn to recognize these five killers and know how to eliminate them, look out! Nothing can hold you back; you're on the road to everything you want. Our next chapter is all about recognizing and remedying these consistency killers so they never slow you down again!

KEY TAKEAWAYS, ACTIONS, AND JOURNAL PROMPTS

As you go through this book, you'll understand that I believe fitness begins in our heads. When you have a fitness mindset, you will find it easier to follow through on your dreams, goals, and vision for your health and your life. Approach these questions with curiosity. We are not here to beat ourselves up, we're here to raise ourselves up to begin living the life we have always dreamed of. Bonus points if you start right now by creating a freedom journal and begin recording your journey. This will come in very handy when you start tracking your fitness steps! The fact that you're here tells me a lot about you, and I'm so glad we're on this journey together!

- *Notice: Where are you putting everyone else and everything first before prioritizing your fitness and personal care?*

    Almost universally, busy women learned early in life to take care of everyone and everything else first. Then, if there was time left over, it was ours. It's time to recognize where you constantly put others first, even if it seems that it is the right thing to do. When we recognize where and how we prioritize others, we can put our creativity to work by asking ourselves, "If I had the time and wherewithal to focus on my fitness, how might that look?"

- *Notice: What currently hurts physically, and how are your energy levels?*

    Do you wake energized and then wear down during the day? Or do you wake up tired and stay that way? Are your joints achy in the morning or the evening? Pay attention. More energy and less pain are some of the first things a client tells me they want, but then they forget to track their energy and pain levels and don't even notice how much better they feel until I ask them! Pay attention; you'll be shocked at how much better you feel very quickly.

- *Notice: How often do you say you'll start next week, only to see that another week just flew by? That hurts. Or, as my client Debbie used to say:*

    "I'll start tomorrow, but I suddenly realized that the date {tomorrow} has never shown up on my calendar, :) I have to act now." Debbie

CHAPTER 3
THE FIVE CONSISTENCY KILLERS

In our heads, the clock is ticking. There's a fear swirling around that we have to make up for all the lost time when we didn't do what we probably should have been doing...eating better, moving more, and taking time for ourselves. Like the white rabbit in Alice in Wonderland, we mutter, "I'm late. I'm late," and there's not a minute to waste. STOP. Take a breath and remember, fitness is a long game. You have time; all you need is awareness! Kelly Howard

Before you can stay on track, you need to recognize what keeps throwing you off track! There are five factors that typically stop our forward momentum, and I like to call them the consistency killers. When we know these potential pitfalls, they are easier to avoid or eliminate.

Awareness Is Key

Take a quick moment to acquaint yourself with these consistency killers so you can recognize when you catch yourself doing them and course correct! They are easy to change when you're aware of what they are.

Consistency Killer #1: Perfection

When something has to be perfect, and it isn't, we quit because we believe that by not being perfect, we have evidence that what we're doing isn't going to work. Perfection isn't natural, and what little bit we can create never lasts. Perfection often begins when we make a plan, and it might be slightly more than we think we can do, but by gosh, it's time to make this fitness thing happen, right??

There will be times that we are kicking butt and taking names, but then life sneaks up on us. Maybe you need to work late, or perhaps you need to take care of somebody or something else. Suddenly you're derailed. Instead of losing sleep or worrying about what you missed or didn't do, you simply bring yourself back on course.

If you find that no matter what you do, you never seem to be able to keep up with your plan, you may need to revisit your plan. In later chapters, you will learn more about creating the perfect plan for you, but here's a good rule of thumb. If you are hitting your plan 80-90% of the time, you're on track and doing great. If you're achieving your plan 100% of the time, it is probably time to revisit and revise your plan; it is probably too easy for you.

A good rule of thumb to keep yourself on track and doing your best is to ask yourself: How important is having your perfect workout, the perfect diet, or even the right amount of calories that you burn daily on a scale of one to ten? Ten being perfection is paramount, the ideal workout and diet is the golden key. One is that the perfect workout and diet are not important at all. What's your number?

After working with thousands of busy, successful women – I have learned that striving for *perfection derails us faster than anything else.* If you can accomplish 80% of your fitness plan, you're on a perfectly sustainable path. Perfection never lasts.

Pattie - went out for lunch with friends and enjoyed a beer, and then when she got home, she didn't feel like doing her afternoon workout. At one point, something like this would have thrown her into a tailspin; all the fear and the stories about "this never works, I never stick to my plan" would have come up. Instead, she simply forgave herself and started back on track the next day. No drama, no worry, just a reset and restart. Life happens, and how we handle it is what matters most. Not the fact that we missed a day.

Consistency Killer #2: Not Anticipating Roadblocks

Roadblocks are anything that throws you off your fitness plan. They can be physical, like travel, work projects, visitors, weather, or holidays. Or you may be in a psychological quagmire where you don't find enough motivation to keep you going. Usually, when it's a physical roadblock, you can plan in advance for it. You'll learn to create your fitness plan around these expected obstacles. For now, just know that when creating your fitness plan, you need to be aware of potential obstacles and be ready to work around them.

But what about the unexpected roadblocks? It could be too much work outside the norm, injuries, poor sleep, or you just don't feel up to moving that day. Maybe you aren't getting the outcomes you desire fast enough. The mental roadblocks are the tough ones. When one of these raises its ugly head and slows you down, see it for what it is. Nothing more than a roadblock. When you miss a day or two, that's all that happened; you missed a day or two. Do not let this derail you!

Roadblocks happen, and then we continue. Done. Sometimes we forget that changing our bodies takes time. Getting our bodies back can take more time than we expect. Dig in and keep going.

Anticipate and accept them. Don't believe you'll be perfect every day (see killer #1:). Don't believe you'll exercise when someone visits if you've never done it before. Life has peaks and valleys when we slip into a valley, take a day off, and then simply restart.

Consistency Killer #3: Going Beyond Your Tipping Point

In Malcome Gladwell's excellent book *The Tipping Point*, he describes the tipping point as **the magic moment when behavior becomes viral and spreads like wildfire**.

I've come to understand there's a different *"Tipping Point"* when it comes to our fitness; *it's that one extra action we add to our plan that stops everything.* It could be that you're humming along with a plan that has you doing cardio thrice a week, resistance twice a week, and some quick mobility a few days per week, and suddenly you decide to add HIIT before your resistance to work on that stubborn fat. It could be a good idea or not, but if it's the one additional action that is too much for your body or your time allotment, you'll find your overall forward momentum coming to a stretching halt.

I've seen this happen in my life more than once regarding supplements. I might have my protein powder and supplements set up, taking them 80-90% of the time. But then I read that I really should add this "one supplement" that will make everything work better…you might know the drill. The problem is this one supplement is the size of a horse pill, and I need to take three to achieve the desired results. So I end up not taking any of my supplements because I don't want to deal with that particular one. I get overloaded with good intentions and stop myself in my tracks.

When we're overloaded, we're trying too hard. We try to do everything possible because we so desperately want to change.

Unfortunately, when we over-commit, something has to give. We hit a roadblock, and it all crumbles.

If you feel overwhelmed by your goals or the schedule you've created, stop and take a step back. Ask yourself, if this was easy, what would you do differently? Go back to scheduling. Go back to your non-negotiables. Grab a tool from your toolbox (you'll learn all about these techniques in coming chapters) and ask yourself, "What do I need to do just a little differently?"

When we give ourselves breathing room, we stop feeling overwhelmed. Everything is easier and starts working again. Remember to do your stuff, but don't do too much of it.

Consistency Killer #4: The All-or-Nothing Mentality

This killer is similar to overloading yourself but is slightly insidious. This is the belief that if you aren't doing it ALL; the exercise, the diet, the weights, the cardio, yoga, and meditation, then what you're doing isn't worth doing. It's the belief that you have to start strong, stay strong, go big, and do it all. *The underlying belief is that you must make up for all the lost time - right now!*

As effective as this might sound, the problem is it's not sustainable, especially for busy women! When you're on this path, and you miss a day, you'll get overwhelmed thinking about all the time and effort it will take to catch up. If you miss a week, well…you might as well give up because it's apparent this isn't going to work for you. You can't stick to this, so why bother?

This is a tough one because when we're superwomen, we're used to doing "all the things." This is your chance to pull back and focus on what you can do now and what matters most. We'll work more on determining what matters most when you create your plan in Part 2.

Consistency Killer #5: Your Personal Kryptonite

The last consistency killer is an interesting one – I call it our Kryptonite. *Kryptonite is the thing, the action, the mindset, or the block that holds us back from everything that we want.* We all have it. It's the consistency killer that we all know we have but pretend it's either not there or not a problem.

Kryptonite can be a physical habit like eating too much sugar or drinking too much wine. It could be a belief we've been dragging around about ourselves for too long. It can be something we need to quit doing or start doing but fear we never will, something that makes us feel secretly embarrassed or weak for even having the issue. It could be a simple habit like surfing social media instead of getting a good night's sleep. It's everywhere.

Whether it is emotional, physical, a long-standing habit, or something that holds us back from what we desire, Kryptonite is a killer.

Everyone has some form of Kryptonite in their life, and it can be a complete game-changer when you're willing to look! The easiest way to uncover your Kryptonite is to just observe precisely what you're thinking it could be right now, at this moment. This is usually where to start.

If you're unsure, ask yourself this question: What are you doing or not doing in your life right now that is stopping you from having the fitness and health you desire?

And then trust your answer.

Fit is Freedom Friend - Dana

My 1:1 client Dana wanted to get leaner and stronger for a series of bike races she had signed up for, but nothing we were doing was truly moving the needle on the scale or the measuring tape. The weight wasn't budging, and her cycling wasn't improving. I knew her food intake, and we were tracking her workouts, but she wasn't sleeping well and was groggy in the mornings. Somewhat baffled, I asked her the Kryptonite questions: *"Is there something you are doing or not doing that you secretly know is holding you back?" "What's the biggest block to your fitness right this minute? What's the one thing that if you change, everything else will change. Tell me the first thing that comes into your mind."*

Somewhat sheepishly, she said, *"I'm drinking too much wine. Most nights, I'm having 2 or even 3 glasses of wine."*

The moment I heard it, I burst into laughter. *"Yep, that might be affecting your sleep, your weight, and your training – LOL."* I was laughing not because I thought she was silly but because I understand how kryptonite makes us do things we know are affecting us determinately, but we pretend otherwise. The problem was, she and her husband enjoyed good wine, and most evenings, when she intended to have just one glass, lively conversations and delightful dinners kept them going, making it hard for her to stop. In fact, she was afraid that if she stopped drinking wine completely, it would make her husband uncomfortable, and anyway, she enjoyed it. Another concern she had was the fear that quitting drinking would mean quitting forever, which wasn't something she was ready to do.

We're all different. Sometimes the kryptonite we experience truly is something we need to eradicate from our lives. Sometimes we get into a habit and just need to hit the pause button and allow ourselves to start fresh.

For Dana, she decided to eliminate the wine for 30 days. After the first 30 days, she decided that drinking during the week wasn't serving her, so she was able to make a lifestyle change that allowed her to still enjoy great wine with her husband on the weekends and, at the same time, make time for herself and her health during the week.

Fit is Freedom Friend - Cindy

Cindy was a single mom who was always low on energy. She felt unmotivated and told the Fit is Freedom Group that she was beginning to feel like every day was getting worse than the day before. Her predicament was wearing her down. I wanted to run her through the Kryptonite Q's but needed to ensure she was okay sharing on a group call.

She said, "Absolutely, I want to figure this out!"

The Fit is Freedom group is a very safe place, a community of women who care and want to see each other succeed. Luckily she felt safe because her answer embarrassed her.

We didn't go any further than the first question: What is the biggest thing holding you back from your fitness dreams?

"My kids" was what came out of her mouth, and she looked shocked and chagrined! Admitting that was tough, but she was willing to do whatever she needed to start feeling better. The truth was, day after day, she would get the kids ready for school in the morning, go to her very busy job, work hard all day, come home, and take care of all the needs of her family, put the youngest to bed numerous times and then when it was her time, she would crash. Her life was always about caring for everyone else. She had no time or energy for herself at the end of the day. She desperately wanted to start exercising again – maybe even do a little reading and relaxing – but she didn't feel like she could because of her obligations to her kids. Any spare time felt like it should be kid time!

After we chatted, she started realizing that putting everyone else's needs before her own did nothing but wear her out, which meant she wasn't really 100% there for her family. She committed to giving herself permission to take time for herself. She started going to pilates three times a week, and her kids figured out how to pitch in and live without her for a couple of hours a week. Just that little bit of exercise made her feel better. Sleep better. Helped her start to make food choices that supported her (the old cascading effect of good in full swing!).

As she felt more empowered, she took more action. Her secret resentment started fading, and she found guilt-free ways to begin caring for herself. She was happier and more fun to be with for the kids. As she worked on removing her Kryptonite, her energy levels rose, and her motivation came back.

One little question allowed these women to make changes that worked; now it's your turn. What's your kryptonite? What is the biggest thing holding you back from your fitness dreams?

When you ask yourself this question, there will be one thing that you immediately think of, and that's it. Don't edit it.

What's the thing that maybe you have tried to change but failed numerous times?

Find out what your kryptonite is and make it a priority to change. Kryptonite is like a giant domino. When you push that domino, all the other things fall into place.

Take Cindy, for example. She told her family that they were just going to have to live without her for three hours a week. And it turned out fine. Once she did that, everything else started falling into place. For Dana, she decided, "What the hell, I'm just going to quit drinking wine 80% of the time for the next 90 days." And she did. She lost weight and started feeling better. She did her bike race and then decided that she liked the change so much that she wanted it to be how she lived her life most of the time.

Your kryptonite doesn't have to be something you quit for the rest of your life. But you need to figure out what's holding you back. After all the years I've worked with people, I have found the key to kryptonite – you don't have to change it or remove it from your life altogether, you just have to shift it a little bit. Push that domino over, and everything else starts falling into place.

Action time! Grab your Fitness Journal, and let's start uncovering your consistency killers. You may only have one, or you might give rein to more; either way, it's time to see where those subtle sabotages are in your life. Move on to the next page and do your exercise.

EXERCISE #2: RECOGNIZING AND AVOIDING CONSISTENCY KILLERS

When it comes to the consistency killers, awareness is key. Journaling will help. Paying attention to what you say to yourself when things are going sideways - this is when awareness will matter most.

Below, rate yourself on a scale of 1-5, 1 being "not accurate at all" and 5 being "most accurate." Total your score and use the answer key to determine your next steps.

Track-it:

- I never worry if I skip my workouts because I know I'll be back on track in no time.
- I believe in intuitive eating; I trust that I'll eat exactly what works for my body and fitness.
- I trust my body to know what needs to be done each day.
- Understanding my kryptonite and banishing it sounds rather fun.
- I'm fine with the idea of only losing a pound a month.
- I've never worried about losing weight for a special event; I am who I am.

- I'm ok with the idea that my workout schedule is just a suggestion.
- I believe that the right fitness plan is exactly what I need to reach my fitness goals.

What your score means:

- **Score 10 - 25**

  One of the most challenging things about consistency killers is that they are things we've been told but in reverse! How many times have you heard that you have to "do it no matter what?" Are you watching your sugar intake, but you have company coming into town? Don't stop your diet. It will ruin everything, your friends can skip desserts! Did you miss two days of your workout plan this week? WTH, aren't you committed to this? Life happens. And life is too short to cut out the things that matter. Do you skip a workout to have beers with your girlfriends? So what? Start over tomorrow. Do you worry that if you aren't all in, then you're all out? I believe in you and know that the more you follow the Fit is Freedom Formula throughout this book, the more awareness you bring to your fitness plan, the more you will shine! You're in the right place, and we'll have fun together!

- **Score 26 - 40**

  Awareness is key, and you have it! Now, it's time to begin focusing on what will move you forward, not what might have held you back in the past. Consistency killers are nothing more than awareness motivators. Look for them, pat yourself on the back when you find that you're falling for them, and then keep moving forward. You, my friend, have got this!

- **Score 41 - 50**

    You have an excellent awareness of what truly holds people back from fitness consistency. I imagine that once you work through the next chapter and then focus on the long game, you'll find creating and following your customized plan a breeze.

KEY TAKEAWAYS, ACTIONS, AND JOURNAL PROMPTS

Consistency killers are never something you need to avoid or stop completely, awareness is key in these situations. Remember, when you have a fitness mindset, you will find it easier to follow through on the dreams, goals, and vision you have for your health and your life. Use curiosity and awareness, not rules and requirements. We are here to live the life we have always dreamed of. Enjoy.

- *Notice: When you feel the need to have perfection…red flag!*

   What do you criticize yourself the most about? Where are you deeply dissatisfied about in your life? How would you feel if you could trust yourself to quit trying so darn hard? Is that scary? Awesome - start there. None of this needs to be perfect. Just do your best in the moment.

- *Notice: What roadblocks seem to stop you from what you want to do and achieve?*

   When you feel like you're hitting roadblocks, take a breath, slow down, and rearrange your fitness/food/life schedule to fit the current roadblock. This is not a long-term change, it's a quick fix for the current environment. Also, look ahead. We often know what is coming our way; schedule for it. Don't just hope it won't be a problem! Is your partner having a medical procedure? You're going to have less time or need to schedule help. Are you traveling, having visitors, or adopting a new puppy? Plan accordingly. Remember, fitness is a long game. Take it week by week and day by day if that's what you need to do in the moment.

Where are you feeling overwhelmed? Have you hit your tipping point and kept trying?

Your fitness is a long game. If you feel overwhelmed by your fitness goals and by the schedule you've created, or whatever it is that you have decreed that you must do, stop and take a breath. Take small consistent steps. When we feel overwhelmed, life seems harder. Remember to stop and breathe, it will work out and it's easier when we're not stressed!

- *Notice: Want to push a big domino over? Use the Kryptonite questions:*

  Is there something you are doing or not doing that you secretly know is holding you back? What's the biggest block to your fitness right this minute? What's the one thing that, if you change it, everything else would change? Write down the first thing that comes to your mind.

"I was so afraid that if I quit drinking wine that meant that I could never enjoy another glass in my life! I realized that when I faced my wine Kryptonite, it lost a lot of the power and I could start making decisions based on what I wanted, not what I was afraid of. This was a deal changer for me!" Dana

CHAPTER 4
YOUR NORTH STAR

> *"If I'm 100% honest, on our first call, when Kelly wanted me to talk about why I wanted to focus on my fitness instead of creating my workout plan immediately, I thought I had made a mistake. I didn't need to TALK, I needed to ACT. The funny thing is, that first call has made a bigger impact on my health and fitness than anything else we have done together. Whenever I'm faltering, off track, or just plain unmotivated, I come back to my **Fitness Why** that we uncovered, and everything starts to flow again." -Sue*

Starting with your Fitness Why

There is a general school of thought that people either move towards pleasure or move away from pain. When it comes to fitness, most of us are moving away from pain. The weight gain, the achy joints, the way we look in our clothes, the way we feel in our skin. Maybe we have less energy than we used to, or we're starting to believe that our age might be more than just a number.

There are so many things that can kickstart the desire to get into shape once and for all. But motivation wanes, and willpower runs out. In fact, if willpower worked, we wouldn't be having this conversation. Willpower is a limited resource. Especially if we're low on energy or the right fuel! We believe that we just aren't motivated enough. If we had enough desire, we could make the changes we want.

This is true and not true. It's not that you don't have enough drive or motivation, it's that you don't have the right kind of motivation.

- Your doctor told you your numbers were off, and you needed to make a change.
- You have an important wedding coming up, and you want to look your best.
- Sweatpants have become your wardrobe staple.
- You're not sleeping, and you'd like to have a date in the next five years!
- Your birthday is coming up, again.

These are all legitimate reasons, but they're not very exciting and not sexy in the least. We need to be thrilled, have things to look forward to, and live well instead of worrying about what's not working or what's lurking around the corner.

Enough of not-good-enough.

Instead of moving away from what's not working, it's time to move toward what you truly want. To create a vision that gets your attention. It's time to get your brain and heart onboard! What will being fit and feeling amazing mean to you? More life in your life? More energy and confidence, more quality time with those you love? More freedom? Being able to do things you've only dreamt of? To be a role model for your kids or grandkids?

Fitness Trainer and reality TV superstar Jillian Michaels speaks out about this frequently. She is known for reminding people that "getting slim for a wedding could be nice, but you'll put it all back on later if you don't have a bigger WHY."

My mom was my larger-than-life role model, and I truly believe I wouldn't be where I am today without her presence in my life. At age fifty, she made the courageous decision to leave a bad marriage and divorce my father. For most of my childhood, she would wake up very early every morning, long before the rest of the house stirred, and practiced yoga. This was back in the '70s when yoga was still on the fringe! Without instructional videos to follow, she relied on LP records, listening attentively and mimicking the pose descriptions. Later, I recall her using yoga magazines as her guide, and eventually, she started teaching classes herself. Remarkably, she continued to teach yoga well into her 80s until she, unfortunately, suffered a stroke.

Beyond the yoga, and once divorced, she wanted something new to do and took up Taekwondo, inviting me to one of her early classes. We were the only women in the class, so they paired us up to spar. Here I am, standing across from my smaller-than-me mom as they demonstrate how to toss someone to the ground. I'm horrified. No way am I going to throw my mother down to the ground! I paused, she sensed weakness, and the next thing I knew, I was flat on my back with the wind knocked out of me and my 118-pound mom smiling from ear to ear.

That woman was dangerous, I never went back!

All kidding aside, what I saw over the next several years was my mom falling in love with Martial Arts and progressing through belt after belt until she was a 5th-degree black belt, a true Master.

I asked her one time why? Why was she doing all this? Her answer was as simple as it was complex.

"I started out wanting to lose weight and look better. I came to realize that I didn't ever want to feel weak or at the mercy of anyone else ever again. From there, it's grown into me loving being strong and powerful, appreciating my body and everything I can do. And I like throwing men around."

I told you she was dangerous. :)

For me, my why is as simple and complex as my mom's. At one level, I just want to wake up feeling great, having all the energy I want and need to do everything I love to do for as long as I'm here on earth.

On another level, I love playing outdoors on all levels. I love hiking, strolling through the woods, or tackling big, hard trails. Backpacking. Cycling. Kayaking, especially whitewater kayaking. All of these things require me to be strong, flexible, energetic, mindful, and able to play really hard, at the top of my game.

And then there's the idea of freedom. Freedom is different for each of us, but at its core, it's being able to live life on your own terms, physically, mentally, and emotionally. To have physical freedom for the long term, we need to care for our health today. Freedom is one of my driving core values. To me, it means living life fully and full-out. From leading an adventure retreat to embarking on a private expedition and enjoying amazing company at a delicious dinner, it all feels like freedom to me. Fitness is definitely one of the paths to freedom for me. It all works together.

What about you? How is your motivation different?

Once you uncover your fitness Why, if you find your motivation waning or you're tempted to ignore your workout plan, you will have a North Star to pull you back on track. In all my years of working with clients, one thing always rings true: Those women who can connect their fitness Why to their dreams are the women who stay on track and get back on track. Every single time. When you attach your fitness goals to the things that touch your heart the most, you'll win every single time.

Find Your North Star

Ready to dive in and connect with your North Star? Grab your Freedom Journal and take a few minutes to answer these questions:

>Why am I doing this fitness consistency thing?
>
>Why do I want to change?
>
>What is a WHY that gets me excited?
>
>What is a WHY worth waking up for?

And then, take those answers and turn them into a positive desire:

>*Because I'm so unfit* **becomes** *because I'm going to be able to do the things I want to do or want to learn to do*
>
>*Because I'm losing muscle and bone* **becomes** *because I'm getting stronger*
>
>*Because I need to lose weight* **becomes** *because I am ready to feel vibrant and good about my body and health*
>
>*Because I'm feeling old* **becomes** *Because I am ready to feel energetic and excited*

Whatever your reason - focus on moving toward what you want to be rather than away from what you don't want.

Fit is Freedom Friend – Ammie

When Ammie and I first started working together, the only "why" she had was her fear of the future. She never had children, her sister had passed away many years before, and she lived alone. She was consumed by the worry of what would happen to her. What would she do if she became ill? She had gained weight, her cholesterol was higher than it should be, and she had never been active. At 62, her future scared her, and all she could see was the possibility of becoming more unhealthy with each passing year. Her "why" was simply how to avoid the grim reality she had imagined lying before her.

I explained to her that our bodies are resilient as long as we give them what they need!

We started with a simple walk plan with a lightly weighted vest and Tai Chi. By adding a lightly weighted vest, she felt more powerful, that she was doing something that would make a big difference. And physically, it was helping her bone strength. We both knew that the small amount of weight she was using wouldn't be a game-changer, but it was a game-starter! She was changing her mindset and her outlook to a place she could grow from.

I added Tai Chi to her plan because it was something that appealed to her (if it's not fun, it's not sustainable), plus it is great for balance, something she was very concerned about.

More than her movement plan, our big focus began with her mental game. I wanted her to escape the fear of the future and enter a place where she had things to look forward to. Where her "why" was no longer survival but thriving!

She pondered the "why" questions. How would she feel if she wasn't afraid of the future? What would she be doing? What would she like to try, experience, or do?

So I asked her, what words would you like to use to describe yourself and your life?

"Crickets." I finally got a text after the first week with one word. Hopeful.

Good start! We met again, went over what she was doing, and spoke a little more about her "why." The next day I received a text with three words: "Dance. Travel. Pain-free."

Brilliant! These were desires we could work with. We went from single-word texts to emails that were excerpts from her journal, and what I saw was more hope and less fear. I saw excitement, possibilities, and new interests.

Today, she is doing amazingly. She's focusing on living life, not fearing what's coming next. When she has injuries or isn't pain-free, she has learned to come back to her "why" and not fall into a funk or fear. In one of her journal entries, she wrote that she had always wanted to travel to Europe by train, "luxury train of course," she wrote. She found a friend who wanted to go, booked her trip, and texted me a photo of her train tickets.

She went from "hopeful" to touring Europe on a luxury sleeper train. I would say her 'why' gave her wings! There is a fantastic amount of power in a simple shift of what we say to ourselves.

> *"I'm making plans to do things I never thought I would do. I've gone on an all-woman hiking trip, I've signed up for a hike and boat adventure, and I'm taking my three grandkids along. My adult kids are like, "Who is this woman," and my husband is just grateful he can sit on his butt while I go play with new friends - LOL!" Suzanne*

Your turn, grab your Freedom Journal and go through the following exercise. Time to find and follow your North Star!

EXERCISE #3: LIVING LIFE IN FULL COLOR

Think about the prompts below and write your thoughts in your Freedom Journal.

1. *Uncover your WHY.*

Who will you be as you master your own fitness consistency? An athlete, a teacher to others, someone enjoying life to the brim? What does embodying being fit feel like to you? **What will being fit feel and mean to you? More life in your life? More energy and confidence, more quality time with those you love?**

2. *Create your Passion Plan.*

To me, the idea of a "bucket list" is constricting. It's like, here are the things I want to do, and then I can just die…Forget that! What if, instead, you start creating an ongoing Passion Plan? Things that you want to do, try, and experience. Knowing that as you experience one thing, it might take you in an entirely new direction! Let's make life a journey filled with new adventures and explorations. It's time to craft a vision of your deepest desires and journeys you've only dreamed of. All of it. **Who you'll be playing with, where you will be, things you'd like to try, and things you thought were in your past but just might be possible, list them all.**

3. *Capture the feelings.*

How do you want to feel in life? What are two words that describe the feelings for this next half of your life? When you think of being as fit as you want to be, how does it FEEL to you? Physically, emotionally, mentally, deep down in your heart, how will you feel? **Feelings are the secret sauce to moving forward. How do you want to feel?**

KEY TAKEAWAYS, ACTIONS, AND JOURNAL PROMPTS

- *Notice: If you could have anything and everything you want physically, what would it be?*

  Forget about "looking good" or the scale for just a minute and dream with me. What will being fit allow you to do? Where will you travel? Who will you take with you? What will you experience?

- *Notice: What are those secret or not-so-secret worries that haunt you? What worries are you willing to let go of for good?*

  Take a moment and thank your body for what it does for you and what it allows you to do.

- *Notice: When you have your own wings, what will you do?*

  Before we're ready for that fun, fit, and free life, we need to address the myth of the quick fix. We live in a society that loves instant solutions. Quick fixes might seem attractive, but they seldom last. In the next chapter, we'll look at why we fall for these options, and you'll learn how to replace a temporary fix with a long-term solution.

CHAPTER 5
FITNESS - THERE ARE NO SHORTCUTS

> *"There are no fitness shortcuts, but that never stops us from hoping."*
> *- Kelly*

Before we begin to uncover the best fitness consistency plan for you, a little tough love. Repeat after me: There are no quick fixes when it comes to our health. So please quit looking.

You're not alone if you've ever fallen for the myth of the magical transformation. It's everywhere we look; lose 30 pounds in 30 days, get sexy arms in two weeks, eat this one spice and lose fat while you sleep. It's hard not to fall for these myths, we're busy, and it would be so much easier if we could just find that alluring fix-all!

It's not your fault! Clickbait is alive and well.

Still, we're smart women, and we've been around long enough to know that when it comes to lasting, sustainable change – quick fixes don't work, you need permanent change, not a bandaid.

Deep down, we all know this. We may advise our friends to 'take it slow, give it time.' Great advice for someone else, yet so unacceptable when talking to ourselves!

Do you secretly think you're the exception to the rule? You're not alone, believe it or not, everyone secretly believes that the rules don't exactly apply to them.

Like the story I told about myself earlier, I secretly believed that my body could magically do everything it needed to do to stay in shape and healthy. All the while, I was doing everything that breaks a body down; sitting for hours on end, eating for comfort instead of fuel, sleeping poorly, doing zero mobility, swimming in Cortisol, and then pushing my physical limits on the weekend. Hmmm, sounds like someone who didn't believe that the rules applied to her!

The only path to lasting success in fitness is to start a little easier than you want to, follow your plan, and stay consistent. This flies in the face of so much advertising and social media's 'go big or go home' messaging. Still, the fact remains that when we can make our fitness repeatable and easy to follow, we have something that works.

Is it sexy? Nope. Will it work for you? Every. Single. Time.

The plan we will put together for you in Part 2 doesn't need to be hard, complicated, or even expensive. You'll find Fit is Freedom Formula to be one of the easiest, most inexpensive, and most manageable exercise concepts you'll ever come across – and that's the point!

Over the next few chapters, we'll work together to develop your fitness consistency plan and uplevel your mindset.

New clients often come to me in a bit of a panic. They have suddenly begun to realize that they're at a point in life where focusing on their fitness is no longer simply a good idea; it's an absolute requirement if they want to live life to the fullest. Changing how they approach fitness is the only thing that will change the trajectory of their life.

Most likely, we'll all live for a fairly long time, medical science can almost guarantee that. But it's up to us to determine how fit and healthy our life will be. Are we going to live vibrant, exciting, adventure-filled lives? Or, will we fade into the background, feeling like hell, unable to do what we want to do as our world slowly shrinks around us?

Not on my watch!

Instead of banking on a quick fix, in this book, you learn how to pull together a sustainable and steady plan based on building your fitness, maintaining it, and pushing when you're ready for more! Suddenly the idea of losing thirty pounds is not an end goal but the beginning of so much more.

If you did the work in Chapter 4, you now have a North Star that gets you excited and out of bed in the morning. The next step is learning how to create a solid foundation to get you where you want to be, no matter what is happening around you. You'll start leaving the quick fixes in the past where they belong. Grab your Freedom Journal, and let's take action!

Before you begin any program, you must know where you are currently and have a foundation to build on. I like to break that foundation into three levels; ***Building, Maintaining, and Ready for more.*** As you work through the Fit is Freedom Formula, you'll learn to recognize what stage you're in and know when it's time to change your stage. You won't need a quick fix because you'll know how to move from level to level when you want to uplevel!

The three levels in the Fit is Freedom Formula are:

Level 1: Building

Level 2: Maintaining

Level 3: Ready for more

In the building phase, you're creating a foundation to grow from. You might be starting from scratch, changing what you've been doing, recovering from an injury, or training for a new adventure!

The building phase is exciting because you're trying new things and seeing how much you can do, but you'll learn that you can't always be in a building phase. There are times our bodies need rest, life gets extra busy, and our schedules are thrown off. Travel, holidays, visiting family, projects, life happens.

In the building phase, you'll start learning to embrace rest. It takes rest for our bodies to get stronger. Adding rest time to your schedule could be the hardest thing you master. In the beginning, everyone worries that if they take a rest or two, they won't start again. They'll be back to the 'next week' syndrome. Nothing can be further from the truth. One of the biggest wins you'll have in this stage is when you learn to trust yourself.

The more you lean on your North Star, the easier it is to trust where you want to go. Your next step will be to create a plan using that star as your guide. You're amazing. We're on this path together, and you will be astounded at what you can achieve and the adventures you will have when your heart, mind, and body are aligned. You've got this, use the building stage to create a strong foundation!

Fit is Freedom Friend - Pam

My client Pam came from a background of being a team coach and an athlete. Life, family, work, injuries, thirty busy years, and then we met. To say she wasn't a fan of starting slow and steady would be an understatement, she hated it!

But, she had lost her fitness foundation and needed to go through the building phase for several months to regain what she worried was lost forever. No way. She is one determined woman, and our bodies are resilient.

Here's a text I received as I was wrapping up this book:

"My dream outcome was to be so much healthier, with better eating, have consistent mobility to be more pain-free, and to be more adventurous until the day I pass. I'm pretty much getting there, thanks to you 😄"

Maintenance comes after you have built a strong foundation and are ready to incorporate your fitness lifestyle into your daily life. In the maintenance stage, you'll be creating fitness habits while maintaining your current fitness level. You may catch yourself slowing down a bit but stay in the sweet spot of doing 80%-90% of what you schedule, and you'll learn to manage the maintenance stage. Your fitness habits become **who you are**.

And then, one day, something will trigger a new goal. Maybe you get invited on a hiking trip, or you finally purchase that kayak or SUP you have wanted, or you sign up for a Fun Run or Walk with a friend. This is when you move into the **Ready for More Phase**!

I love whenever someone reaches this stage. No matter the incentive, you'll find that it's time to push a little harder, create a new training plan, or take up a new activity. When you find yourself reaching for new challenges, you might have a moment when you wonder (like my client Sarah texted me), *"Who is this woman I've become* 🖤*?"*

The next thought should be…someone amazing, of course!

As you're moving through each of these stages, one thing to keep an eye out for is anything that takes you off your path or has you feeling like you're slipping backward. This doesn't mean you missed a day or even a week. It's when your fitness slips your mind, and you pretend your schedule doesn't exist! This can happen when you're overwhelmed in life or feel like you can't slow down. You could find yourself derailed by an injury, and instead of Fitness-Flipping (we'll discuss this in a later chapter), you come to a screeching halt.

Keep in mind if you find yourself slipping, don't panic! You've now learned the power of awareness and how to avoid the consistency killers, you have your North Star, and you understand that fitness has stages. You are simply in a particular moment in life, and you'll learn in the next few chapters how to move out of inertia and back into action.

Above all, don't fall for the myths of "next week I'll start again" or even worse... "This isn't for me, it's probably time for me to slow down." I never want you to feel that way again. We're often led to believe that when we get to a certain age that it's time to take it easy, cut back on what we do, and be careful with those joints. Banish those thoughts, ladies!

Remember, fitness is a long game. If you haven't prioritized your fitness for a year, a decade, or even more, it may take a while to get on track. Stay the course, keep moving, our bodies our resilient, and you've got this.

Fit is Freedom Friend – Sharon

I was leading an in-person hike in my hometown of Houston, Texas. A big crowd had gathered in the parking lot, ready to hit the trails. Houston is relatively flat, but the trails that day had quite a few up-and-down areas, not high but definitely steep. It promised to be a fun, increase-your-pulse kind of day.

As we readied to leave, I saw a car pull up to the side, and a lady got out with a cane. People often use hiking poles on my hikes, but I'd never seen someone with a cane before!

I walked over to let her know we'd be leaving shortly, and she said, *"Oh, I'm not going on the hike, that's too much for me. I have bad knees, and they hurt all the time. I just wanted to prove to myself that I would show up. Maybe in a few months, I'll try to join you on an easy hike."*

I appreciated her candor, but I could only believe that if someone took the time to meet us at the trailhead, deep down, she must be hoping she could come along. She deserved the chance to join us on the hike! With lots of cajoling and assurances that she would not slow us down, I convinced her to come along.

She worked hard, and the hike became one of those "it takes a village" moments; everyone was there to help her up and back down the steep slopes, encouraging and cheering her on. It was an amazing show of courage on her part and camaraderie on the part of the hikers.

When we finally finished and got back to the parking area, she was smiling so big it was almost blinding and kept saying, *"Oh my gosh, that was amazing. I never thought I could do something like that. When I told my knee doctor I wanted to start hiking, he said it was a bad idea. I think it's a great idea!"*

We all cheered.

Sharon had a dream. She had always wanted to hike Yosemite, specifically Yosemite Falls Trail. I've done it, and it's not for the faint of heart. In fact, it's one of the harder National Park day hikes, especially when you add in the grueling section of stair-like rocks that seem to go on forever!

Together we worked on her fitness and hiking skills for a little less than a year. Even though she had finished that earlier Houston hike, I suggested that she dial it back and start small. We focused on short walks, lots of mobility work, and simple strength training. As she got stronger and her knees no longer hurt, we added walking up stairs and short hills. After several months of working together and seeing her progress, she decided to move closer to her daughter and grandkids. I didn't hear from her for a couple of years until one day, I got a text with a photo.

There she was, at the trailhead for Yosemite Falls Trail, having just finished the challenging 7-mile hike for her 65th birthday. She'd invited two younger friends to join her, and they had been training for several months. She went on to say that she was taking off to go travel and hike the USA for a year.

Wow, from struggling with a cane in the molehills of Houston to rocking kick-ass hikes around the country, you can say she's living her life fully these days!

Ready to dump the shortcuts and have a fitness plan that works? Grab your Freedom Journal, and let's ensure you aren't relying on useless shortcuts. Complete the exercises given next and then get ready for Part 2. You'll get hands-on help in creating a plan that takes you from where you are today to exactly where you want to be tomorrow.

EXERCISE #4: ELIMINATING THE QUICK FIXES

We live in a society that values speed, getting things done yesterday, and multitasking while we're at it! When our health is just one more thing to check off the to-do list, we don't give it the care and focus it deserves. Below, rate yourself on a scale of 1-5, 1 being "not accurate at all" and 5 being "most accurate." Total your score and use the answer key to determine your next steps.

Having a long-game mentality:

- I never worry that it might be too late to get in shape.
- I have purchased supplements that promise weight loss, and more than once.
- I trust myself to stick to a fitness plan.
- I focus on my overall health more than my weight.
- I schedule play time in my calendar.
- I trust myself to make good food choices.
- I don't worry about my future and my health.
- I never follow fad diets.
- I have plans and adventures to look forward to.
- When I think about the future, I feel great.
- I am willing to do what it takes to have the health and body I desire.
- I trust my body and rest when I need to.

What your score means

- **Score 10 - 25**

  I am so glad you are here! We live in a society that values the quick fix, and you might have jumped on that wagon more than once. But the fact that you are here tells me you're willing to slow down, take steps that will make a difference, and you're ready to change your life. Congratulations, I'm so glad you are here.

- **Score 26 - 40**

  It's time to trust yourself and look forward. You've been taking steps that are putting you on the right path, it's time to fine-tune that plan and stick to it. One step in front of the other and keep reading, this book was written for you.

- **Score 41 - 50**

  You are a rock star, and you are finding new ways to enjoy fun and fitness in this beautiful life. Keep reading for even more ideas to take your fitness to the next level.

Congratulations, you have done amazing work, working through these last five chapters. Give yourself a pat on the back and get ready to create your fitness plan that brings it all together. It's time to go from dreaming and being ready, to doing exactly what needs to be done to create your active and ageless life, for a lifetime!

KEY TAKEAWAYS, ACTIONS, AND JOURNAL PROMPTS

- *Notice: Are you in a rush for your body to change?*

    If you feel like you need to be in a desperate hurry, grab your fitness journal and write out why you feel that way. Once it's on paper and visible, it won't have the hold over you it did in the past.

- *Remember, fitness is a long game.*

    If you haven't been prioritizing your fitness for a year, a decade, or even more, it will take to get on track. But, our bodies are resilient and you're here for the long term!

- *Notice: Are you secretly looking for a quick fix?*

    Are you banking on a quick fix? It is time to learn how to pull together a sustainable and steady plan based on building your fitness, maintaining it, and pushing when you're ready for more. Banish the idea that losing thirty pounds is the goal, start believing that it is the start of so much more.

- *Remember: Clickbait is alive and flourishing!*

    Where have you fallen prey to the idea of the quick fix and where can you make permanent change instead of a bandaid?

PART 2

CHAPTER 6
A LIFE OF FREEDOM BEGINS BY DESIGN

"If consistency is the key, then a well-designed fitness plan is the door that opens to everything you desire!"- Kelly

A funny thing about our health and fitness is that we treat them differently than almost anything else in our lives. We'd never start a major project at work without a plan of action, take a road trip without looking at a map or go to the grocery store without a list. But fitness...it's different! It is treated as something to just fit in where you can, when you can, and only when you have time. The reality is if it's not scheduled, it's not real.

Many of my clients initially struggle with the concept of a structured plan. As one person laughingly said to me, "You and that plan, you aren't the boss of me." She was laughing, but she was also serious. Having so many other responsibilities in her life, a written weekly fitness plan felt like just one more "have to" instead of something to look forward to. You'll learn in Chapter 11 about FPA, but for right this moment, just know - when you learn to plan ahead, not only will you master your fitness and health, but it gets easier too!

One unexpected win almost everyone agrees on is that when they create and stick to their weekly fitness plan (all the details of creating your plan are coming up in the next chapter), they relish the freedom it ultimately gives them. When you have a plan, you quit negotiating with yourself and simply do what needs to be done.

You can then check it off your to-do list for the day, feeling the power of completion. With the right plan, you'll have a clear direction and a roadmap for success.

It's time to create your personal plan!

Fit is Freedom Friend - Shelly

I've known Shelly for years through a business mastermind. She is a fantastic powerhouse – a bright, strong woman taking the business world by storm. Over the years, we would see each other at business events, and every single time, she would tell me the story of her latest fitness strategy. *'This is it, Kelly,'* she would say. *'This is what's going to get me where I want to be.'* She tried everything; I mean everything. Personal trainers, 7 days a week workouts, Pilates, yoga, cross-fit, marathon running, paleo, keto, vegan, intermittent fasting. You name a trend, and I can guarantee you with almost 100% certainty that she tried it.

Over the years, I would cheer her on but never offer my opinion. As much as I liked Shelly, I didn't think she would appreciate my plan-based, start slow and grow slowly approach to fitness. That it doesn't happen overnight and is something you do forever and not just something to do until you hit a number on the scale!

Conversation after conversation, they were always the same – how the latest attempt hadn't worked. Now she was already onto the newest fitness fad du jour, a new start; she'd assure me that this time, it would absolutely work. All the while, I'd be biting my lip. Not one to give unsolicited advice. She had this intense, all-or-nothing approach when it came to changing her health that simply wasn't sustainable.

Finally, defeated after injuring herself while training for a marathon, when she had never been a runner before, she said, "Kelly, I'm starting to feel like it might be time to give up, to throw in the towel. Nothing I try seems to work. I just keep gaining and losing the same weight. I'm in pain and feel like I'm too old to accomplish my fitness goals.

Is there anything you can do to help me?"

"Shelly' I said. 'The thing is, if we're going to do this, we're going to do it my way — and trust me, you're not going to like my way at first, but if you stick with the plan we create, I promise you will see the results that you've been chasing after for so many years!"

She was desperate, and she agreed. We began working together, but boy, she fought me at the start. The first week of her plan started out simple but with a purpose; a brisk, 30-minute daily walk and some simple mobility work to get her joints healthy and her body moving again. I had her track what she ate, but she could eat whatever she wanted to.

'A Walk?' she texted me when I first sent her the simple plan. *'A WALK!?!'*

She was incredulous. *'How am I going to get in shape and lose weight walking? Plus, I need a food plan. I don't trust myself to eat whatever I want to eat. I'll just gain weight.'*

After years of diet upon diet and extreme workouts, her body needed a rest and a reset. Begrudgingly she did the first week and then the second. We built her workout plan from there. She began to trust herself; what to eat, how to move, when to push harder, and when to slow down. Slowly but surely, we added more movement and different foods. Her fitness and self-care became a habit instead of a fad, and her routine became a part of who she is, a strong, fit woman. There were times she was annoyed to no end because, to her, a person who was used to an all-or-nothing approach, it felt like she was moving way too slowly.

Except it wasn't too slow – once we had a foundation in place and she started building consistent fitness habits, the results began to show. Around month three, she was beginning to realize that not only did she have the habits of an athlete, but she was also no longer flailing about for the next best thing. She started to relax and enjoy her workouts. She was wearing pants that she hadn't worn in years. Her energy levels, diet, and weight were naturally where she wanted them to be, and she was sleeping well. All because of the small, consistent, and incremental changes she made on a daily basis.

What I saw was someone who had started trusting herself. Who had things to look forward to that didn't revolve around what the scale said. She was making plans and enjoying life instead of being afraid of what might come next. She was no longer searching for that magic 'thing' outside herself; she was living it. Shelly was embracing a fit and free life for possibly the first time ever.

Ready For Your Plan?

- Truth: There are thousands of cookie-cutter "workout routines" in the world.
- Truth: You wouldn't be reading this book if they worked!

Let me tell you another story of one of my amazing clients, Andrea. Andrea, joined us after realizing that she'd been going to the gym for over six months with zero results. Absolutely no body composition change! Even worse, she had aches and pains that she had never had before. She was despondent. Three days of her life every week at a gym she didn't like and no results to show. She was ready to throw in the towel and grab the remote!

Several months later, she told me that following the Fit is Freedom Formula changed her life, mind, and body. But what was behind such a drastic change? The fact that she took the time to understand everything that needed to be included in her fitness plan. And then, she took the time to create her own plan and revise it when needed. She learned what she likes and what she doesn't. Life is too short to do things that don't light us up, especially when it comes to fitness and health.

The funny thing? Today, two years later, she's back at the gym. Here's the big difference between Andrea today at the gym and Andrea two years ago. After creating and following her own Fitness Freedom Plan, she is now empowered to do what works. She has a personal trainer and has no qualms about telling him if something isn't working or if she doesn't like a particular move. Learning to create her plan empowered her, and it changed her life. When we're empowered, we can do anything.

Ready to achieve the results you want? In the next chapter, you will learn the steps to building your plan, but first, grab your Freedom Journal, and let's figure out where you are on the consistency scale and where your weaknesses might be. This exercise takes just a few minutes and will set you up to win!

EXERCISE #5: SET YOURSELF UP TO WIN

Below, rate yourself on a scale of 1-5, 1 being "not accurate at all" and 5 being "most accurate." Total your score and use the answer key to determine your next steps.

Having a structured fitness plan:

- I currently have a structured fitness plan in place.
- I believe having a structured fitness plan is essential for achieving my fitness goals.
- I find it easy to stick to a structured fitness plan.
- I feel more motivated and empowered when I have a structured fitness plan.
- I have seen positive results from following a structured fitness plan.
- I struggle to stick to a structured fitness plan.
- I feel overwhelmed by the idea of creating a structured fitness plan.
- I believe a structured fitness plan takes away my freedom and flexibility.
- I am willing to make time to create and follow a structured fitness plan.

- I believe a structured fitness plan will help me achieve long-term success and freedom in my fitness journey.

What your score means:

- **Score 10-20:**

    You may not have a structured fitness plan in place or have struggled to stick to one. It's understandable to feel overwhelmed or resistant to the idea, but a structured plan can actually provide more freedom and flexibility in the long run. Consider the benefits and start small by creating a simple plan for the upcoming week.

- **Score 21-30:**

    You understand the importance of a structured fitness plan and have likely seen positive results from following one. While it may not always be easy to stick to, you recognize its value in achieving your fitness goals. Keep up the good work, and consider ways to fine-tune your plan for even greater success.

- **Score 31-40:**

    You are ready and willing to create and follow a structured fitness plan! You understand its importance for achieving long-term success and are willing to make time to prioritize your health and fitness. Keep up the amazing work, and continue to adjust your plan as needed for continued success.

- **Score 40-50:**

    You understand the power of a structured fitness plan and are ready for even more positive results. Keep up the amazing work, and consider sharing your knowledge and experience with others who may benefit from your experiences.

KEY TAKEAWAYS, ACTIONS, AND JOURNAL PROMPTS

- *Stop putting off starting your fitness journey.*

    Many of us say that we will start next week, only to find that another week has flown by. This can be frustrating, but it's important to remember that consistency is key. A written fitness plan can serve as a roadmap to help you achieve your goals and progress toward the life you've always dreamed of.

- *Use habit stacking or habit shifting to change your fitness habits.*

    Changing habits can be tough, but it's easier when you have a plan. Habit stacking involves anchoring one new habit to an existing habit, while habit shifting involves changing or replacing a current habit that doesn't support your goals. Start with small, achievable habits and build from there.

- *Create a structured fitness plan to help you achieve your goals.*

    A weekly written fitness plan can serve as your roadmap to success. Use visual aids, schedule classes, and events, and track your progress in a journal. Focusing on internal support and being gentle with yourself can help you stay on track and progress toward your goals.

- *Journal Prompts: Grab your pen and your freedom journal and answer these prompts.*
- What are some unwanted habits that you want to change, and why?
- How can you use habit shifting or habit stacking to make progress toward your fitness goals?
- What motivates you to prioritize your fitness and personal care?
- What are your current fitness habits, and how can you shift them to better align with your goals?

CHAPTER 7
CREATING YOUR CUSTOM FITNESS PLAN

"The women I work with don't come to me because they want six-pack abs. They come to me because they want to be able to do everything they want to do and do it for a very long time. Of course, the abs are a nice bonus!"- Kelly

The Disclaimer

Remember, in our litigious society, I must remind you to check with a doctor before starting any workout plan. If you have medical issues, please take them into consideration and don't push past what you can and should be doing.

In my own words, use common sense! If you have medical issues, ask your doctor what you can do without causing issues. Next, learn to trust yourself and your body. Always put mobility first; your joints need to be healthy to move well, and remember, pay attention to what your body tells you!

The Preliminaries to Fitness Plan

Workout plans fail if they don't take into consideration YOU. Who you are, the life you currently lead, and your dreams. When everything is based on cookie-cutter, do this and then do that, how can it possibly work for you as an individual? Your body comprises your unique history, lifestyle, injuries, how active or inactive you have been, and what you are willing to commit to. Add to that how much time you have to devote to this, what your body can do, and what you enjoy doing, and the only thing that makes any sense is a personalized plan!

When I work with a new client, we go through a detailed Q&A to make sure:

A. We're starting from the right Level.

B. We look at her current activities and anything she does that she can add to her plan.

C. We look at all the possibilities for mobility, resistance, and cardio. What she likes to do and, even more importantly, what she doesn't like. If it's not fun (to some degree), it will not be sustainable.

D. How much (realistically) time she has to devote to her fitness.

E. We are taking her goals into consideration.

F. For you to follow this same process, you have two choices. You can either use the Client Quiz you will find in the bonuses at www.FitisFreedom.com/bonuses or take the abbreviated quiz below. Once you have your level, make sure it 'feels' right for you. It is always better to start at a lower level and then move up as you feel ready for more. *Remember, starting small is starting smart!*

Once you have your level, next you will pick your mobility, resistance, and cardio options. If you take the online quiz, it will help you choose your options. Otherwise, you'll find numerous options later in this chapter. Be realistic about the time you are willing to devote to this. If you've been inactive and suddenly decide to devote an hour a day, 6 days a week to your plan, do a little soul-searching. Is this really going to happen? Once again, it's better to start small and build up than start big and feel like a failure if you don't hit your goals.

Finally, keep your North Star and all other goals in your mind as you build your plan.

The starting point - You must know your current fitness level

Scale: Give yourself a point for every YES

1. Do you engage in physical activity at least 3 times each week?
2. Would you rate your current level of physical fitness above 5 on a scale of 1-10?
3. Can you walk vigorously for 20 minutes without becoming overly fatigued?
4. Have you maintained your strength, flexibility, and endurance in recent years?
5. Are you currently following any fitness goals or plans?
6. Do you regularly incorporate strength training exercises into your fitness routine?
7. Do you feel confident performing exercises with correct form and technique?
8. Do you regularly incorporate flexibility or mobility exercises into your routine?
9. Do you often feel excessively tired or sore for days after a workout?
10. Have you noticed a positive impact on your mood or stress level after exercising?

Score:

1-4   Level One - Beginner

4-6   Level Two - Intermediate

6 -10   Level Three – Advanced

Note: if you're a 4 or 6 score, you can choose which level you want to create your workout. Also, write your fitness level, whatever it may be, in your Freedom Journal for future reference.

My Suggested Timeframe

Typically, months 1-2 are the experiment stage for my clients. Don't worry about getting it right. Think about trying new things, finding what works for you, and enjoying the process. Frequently, when women work with me, they can be in a bit of a panic, believing they're at the now-or-never stage. Things need to happen fast! During the experiment months, you'll be taking action. It just may not feel like you're moving fast, but you won't believe you've figured it out until you look back later on, especially if you've been tracking your progress! Don't worry about right or wrong, remember, it's an experiment. May I suggest you approach this stage willing to take imperfect action? You can't get it wrong because it's an experiment. You've got this!

Months 2-4 are application time. This is when you apply everything you've learned and start testing new ideas and actions. You'll be putting together weekly plans that build up from the week before or that are designed to maintain the fitness that you now have.

Months 4 and on? This is when you'll truly start seeing progress! All your hard work will pay off, and your fitness consistency will become second nature to you. You'll be refining what you do and possibly training for something special. This is when you find yourself in the Ready for More stage. Remember back in Chapter 5 when I talked about the 3 levels in the Fit is Freedom Formula? This is you applying the levels and taking action. Congratulations!

Fit is Freedom Friend - Cathy

My new client came to me in a panic; she had booked a trip to climb Kilimanjaro, which was coming up in two months. She hadn't been training or doing much of anything, and her fitness was a low level two at best. She wanted a miracle and expected me to show her how to make it happen. Unfortunately, I had to be the one to tell her I didn't think she could do the training or the trip [without injuring herself]; she simply didn't have enough time for her body to get ready. I suggested she check with the outfitter to see if she could change her trip date. Outfitters want people to be at the top of their game, too! Luckily she was able to rebook the trip for 6 months out, and we worked together to get her up that mountain. The photos and the smiles were worth that work, and she finished feeling great, free of any potential injuries.

It takes time to change, and everyone thinks the rules don't apply to them!

What are you currently doing for your fitness?

If you're currently doing something you enjoy, can you add it to your plan? Consider all the areas of your life, who you are and what you love to do, your time priorities, and when you have time to devote to this. Bottom line, how much time are you really willing to put toward starting your fitness journey?

Options And Activities To Choose From For Your Plan:

1. **Mobility**

You need some form of joint and muscle warm-ups. Our bodies have been taking care of us for a very long time, and they have been compensating for everything we do; sitting more than moving, overuse of certain joints and body parts, and ignoring pain signals our body has been giving, sometimes for decades! Most of us grew up thinking we needed to do static stretching. Stretching is important for muscle flexibilty, but you are going to hear me refer to this type of movement as Mobility. Mobility is dynamic movement. Personally, I believe that gentle, slow, dynamic movement is best for our bodies. Mobility & flexibility (static stretching) are often used interchangeably. Here's what you should know: Mobility refers to how a joint moves through its normal range of motion. Flexibility is the ability of a muscle to stretch temporarily. Flexible muscles help improve how well you move your joints, and that's why flexibility is an important component of mobility.

Mobility is the movement of our joints through their full range of motion and it lets us reach high, squat down, or hike down a rocky trail. When our joints are stiff, it's like having rusty hinges, and even simple moves can feel hard and painful. And that's where flexibility comes in - the underlying secret ingredient to maintaining our mobility.

I have found that when I focus on my mobility, I gain in the short term and long term. If I do my mobility moves prior to a long hike, my body feels better throughout the hike and after. Mobility truly matters for how our bodies feel and what we can do.

Here is a partial list of mobility/flexibility options. Don't go down a rabbit hole looking all of these up. Use this as a guide to pick one, possibly two, options to get started. Truly anything that loosens up stuck joints, fascia, and muscles helps. You'll see I've even included massage in this list! Also, in your bonuses, I've included a couple of my favorite mobility videos to get you started.

- Mobility (basic moves) videos in the bonus
- Myofascial techniques like trigger balls and foam rollers

- Massage
- Yoga
- Yin Yoga
- Pilates
- Tai Chi
- Barre
- Stretch Classes
- Aerial Yoga
- Dynamic Stretching
- Physiotherapy
- Bikram/Hot Yoga
- Static stretching

2. **Cardio**

Cardio is often either a love-it or hate-it option. There are ways to learn to love it that we're going to discuss here, but first, a quick note to my cardio addicts (myself included). If you're a cardio addict, you've probably been doing cardio exercises for a long time. In fact, I bet back in your 30's, if you wanted to lose weight, you would just turn up the cardio and lower the calories. It doesn't work that way anymore. Too much cardio burns muscle instead of fat (and you definitely do not want to start losing muscle). It can even increase your weight by producing more cortisol.

Choose one or two options from the list below, ensuring that each activity lasts less than an hour. While you can schedule longer adventure days if desired, keep in mind that the primary objective is muscle building rather than excessive calorie burning. It is recommended to prioritize shorter workouts on most days and reserve longer sessions for specific occasions.

This is a partial list of cardio options. Pick one or two from this list, or add your own and start here.

- Stair workouts (inside stairs, stadiums, and parking garages during inclement weather)
- Hill training
- Biking (outdoor)
- Spin class
- Rowing machine
- House cleaning (high effort)
- Yard work (high effort)
- HIIT
- Running
- Walking
- Swimming
- Hiking
- Rowing
- Dancing
- Elliptical
- Treadmill
- Cross-Country Skiing
- Indoor Cycling
- Water Aerobics

My Own Cardio Story

When the pandemic came to Houston in March 2020, I was enjoying a cycling weekend with my girlfriends. We'd spent three days in the hills of Texas, riding long distances and not paying any attention to the news. We returned to a city (like the rest of the world) in turmoil and fear. Suddenly everything was closed, and the news was dire.

Long weekend rides were common for me and had never been a problem as I also spent at least 3 days each week at the gym lifting. I was in good shape with weight where I wanted it, and muscle to boot.

Suddenly, the world was in an uproar, and we were all in uncharted territory. With the gym closed and my stress levels out the roof, I started riding and hiking almost daily. A lot. For hours I would roam the trails on my own. My stress would lower only to come home to even more dire news and tragedy worldwide.

It was the same for everyone.

It took a few months, but suddenly, I noticed I was gaining weight! With my mind occupied elsewhere, I hadn't put together how the nasty mix of stress and cortisol was affecting me and everyone else I knew. All that cardio and still gaining weight, what the heck? Without really thinking it through, I just took longer rides. Eventually, I came to my senses and realized all that cardio mixed in with the cortisol and little to no resistance training was wearing my body in a way that had never happened before. I was gaining weight, especially around my stomach, and losing muscle. It was time to make drastic changes.

This isn't just my story. It's the story of almost every woman client I have. Those years of 2020 to 2022 put everyone in flight or fight mode, packed on the pounds, and increased muscle loss. If this happened to you, I'd like you to know two things. First, you aren't alone. My typical client gained somewhere between 15-25 those years. Next, your body is resilient, but you need to add resistance training to get back to where you want to be!

3. **Resistance**

Resistance training can traditionally have a bad rap. So many women have been told for years that they must go to the gym thrice a week for an hour, minimum. This is a big problem if you don't like the gym, don't know what to do at the gym, or even don't have a gym in your area! Let me just say there are multiple options for resistance training, BUT you need to do resistance work. You'll find plenty of options to pick from on the list below, but you *must* (I don't use that word lightly). You must add some resistance to your workout plan.

Why is resistance so important?

At about age 30 (give or take), we start losing muscle mass. By 40, bone mass can start dissipating. Both of these issues can be slowed or stopped with resistance training. Plus, muscles increase your metabolism, helping to boost weight loss. They can lower the possibility of chronic diseases through improved metabolic health, improving sleep, and boosting your mood. And they help with plain old functional fitness - how well you move through life!

Don't let old tapes stop you from starting some form of resistance. I promise, just try the different options I've suggested until you hit on the ones that feel right for you. And then, keep going. The more strength you build, the more you will love it!

- Bodyweight Exercises
- Resistance Bands
- Free Weights/barbells
- Weight Machines
- Suspension Training
- Medicine Balls
- Kettlebell Training

- Pilates
- Yoga
- Jazzercise (dance or barbell class)
- Peloton Digital
- Beachbody
- Barre

Fit is Freedom Friend - Kate

In her early 70s, Kate decided to go all in on her fitness plan. She was ready to lose weight, gain muscle and be as active as she wanted to be. Previously, she had done some Pilates and cycling but had gotten away from these for a few years. She joined my 12-week Accelerator Program determined to lose the belly fat she'd gained and get stronger. She got serious with her resistance workouts, adding two to three resistance training per week. Because she loves cardio and has the option of group classes, bike rides, and treadmill workouts, she added in cardio several times per week. She graciously shared an anecdote with us about her volunteer work, which involved the transportation of several large boxes. Anticipating the arrival of a "70-year-old lady" who might require assistance, the group prepared themselves to lift and load the boxes. However, much to their surprise, there was no need for their help. Approaching the scene with the confidence of a tiger, exhibiting excellent posture and a body that moved effortlessly, she singlehandedly tackled the task, leaving the volunteers searching for the "lady in her 70s" who supposedly required assistance.

Adding a Touch of Adventure.

Sometimes you need to push out of your comfort zone and skip the same old movement. I love adding a touch of adventure to my schedule. Weekly when possible, but even occasionally is a great start. Adventure can be anything you'd like to try or is "different" from your usual workouts. This is your chance to pick options outside the box. Options that excite you. One of my favorite exercises with my clients is the Audacious Adventure list. I challenge them to devise a list of 3-8 activities they would like to do or try. Something that pushes them a little past their comfort zone and uses their newfound fitness. Once we stretch ourselves, we never return to the same person we were before. When you're ready to add some adventure days to your plan, here are some options to try!

- Hiking (especially new or harder trails)
- Cycling
- Canoeing/Kayaking
- Outdoor Yoga
- Stand Up Paddleboarding
- Snorkeling
- Horseback Riding
- Photography Walks
- Trail Running
- Pickleball
- Mountain Biking
- Rock Climbing
- Water Skiing
- Surfing
- Rollerblading
- Rowing
- Cross-Country Skiing
- Downhill skiing
- Snowshoeing

- Skating
- Parkour

You have now determined your starting level and have hopefully found a few options in the Mobility, Cardio, Resistance & Adventure lists. All that's left to do before you start creating your own plan is to decide how much time you are willing to give to your fitness plan. I can give you some very general guidelines, but this is up to you. Choosing (and finding) your time frame depends on your lifestyle, willingness to remove time wasters, and ability to find the time you need in your life.

You now have everything you need to start creating your plan. Below you will find details on how to layout your movement options and several real-life example plans from clients. In these example plans, you'll see a description of each client's lifestyle, time allotment, and level they were at. You'll also see how different clients had different issues that they brought to the plan and how we worked with them.

Designing your Month One Fitness Plan

Start with easy, time-appropriate options that fit your current lifestyle. Remember, start small. You can always add more. It can take a little time to create your plan the first few times. As you get better at this, it will get easier and easier until it becomes a two-minute process once a week! Grab your Freedom Journal, and let's get started! Writing by hand, not typing, uses more of our brain, including our RAS (Reticular Activating System) or 'brain gatekeeper.' This helps us focus, follow our North Star, add extra goals, and ignore distractions.

Start with your current fitness level and pick the appropriate number of options from each category. If you are already taking some actions that can be added to your plan that you like, keep them. Don't overload yourself. Make your plan suitable to the available time. Your time for exercise will expand as it becomes easier and more important to you!

Level 1

- **Mobility:** pick up to 2 options from the above lists for a total of 3-4 times per week
- **Cardio:** pick up to 2 options from the above lists for a total of 1-3 times per week
- **Resistance:** pick 1 option from the above lists for a total of 1-2 times per week

Level 2

- **Mobility:** pick up to 2 options from the above lists for a total of 3-5 times per week
- **Cardio:** pick up to 2 options from the above lists for a total of 2-3 times per week
- **Resistance:** pick 1 option from the above lists for a total of 1-3 times per week

Level 3

- **Mobility:** pick up to 2 options from the above lists for a total of 3-5 times per week
- **Cardio:** pick up to 2 options from the above lists for a total of 2-4 times per week
- **Resistance:** pick 1 option from the above lists for a total of 2-3 times per week

Note: Pick your own adventures and add them to your schedule as you have time and space. Also see the sample plans I've included at the end of the chapter, and then have a hand at creating your own!

Building Your Month One Plan!

To give you ideas on how your plan can come together, I've included several clients and the plan that worked for each of them. You'll notice plans are unique to each individual. No mundane, one size fits all plans here! In these example plans, you'll see that everyone started from different fitness levels, and had their own obstacles, unique goals, and dreams.

As you read through these examples, brainstorm a little, and add notes in your Freedom Journal of what sparks your interest, sounds exciting, and activities you have zero desire to try!

Client Example Ginny - Level One

Ginny began at level one, not because she had never been an athlete, but because it had been many years since she was active. In the past, she competed in sprint triathlons, half marathons and lived a very active lifestyle. However, circumstances changed, and Ginny became the caretaker for her father and granddaughter while also working a full-time job. Her busy life took a tremendous toll, resulting in significant weight gain and total energy loss. When we started working together, Ginny realized not only did she need to lose around 50 pounds, her cardio was shot! The former runner could barely sustain a brisk walk for 5 minutes, let alone five miles.

Her first step was to focus on weight loss because this was causing her the biggest worry. She tackled this with the guidance of a doctor and some hefty adjustments to her diet. I suggested making healthier choices when she felt triggered and upset about certain life circumstances.

For her fitness and movement goals, we started small with very gentle daily mobility exercises, recognizing the impact of her years of a sedentary lifestyle on her joints and overall well-being. When evaluating her overall fitness level, it became apparent that she needed to gain muscle and balance, which of course, more muscle would help with. She started with easy resistance training utilizing bands, 2-3 days a week. Since she loved walking so much, I had her walk as many days as she wished, keeping it under 40 minutes and adding a High

Intensity Interval Training session for about 5 minutes twice weekly.

After six months, Ginny had achieved significant progress. She lost approximately 30 pounds and gained visible muscle definition, particularly in her arms and legs. Her transformation was remarkable, and she felt fantastic. With newfound confidence, she turned a couple of her walking days into run training and finished her first 5K in over fifteen years!

PART 2

Ginny's Month One Training Plan:

Monday	Tuesday	Wednesday	Thursday	Friday	Saturday	Sunday
20 Minutes Resistance/ Mobility Meditative, relaxing walk	30 minutes Walking at PE 3	20 minutes Resistance/ mobility 30 minutes walking at PE 2-3 + HIIT walking session 5 minute	Rest day	20 minutes Resistance/ Mobility 30 minutes walking at PE 3	25+ minutes walking at PE 2-3 15 minute HIIT session	Rest day
Monday 20 Minutes Resistance/ Mobility Medatative, relaxing walk	Tuesday Mobility 30 minutes Walking at PE 3	Wednesday 20 minutes Resistance/ mobility 30 minutes walking at PE 2-3 + HIIT walking	Thursday Rest Mobility	Friday 20 minutes Resistance/ Mobility 30 minutes walking at PE 3	Saturday 30+ minutes walking at PE 2-3 15 minute HIIT session	Sunday Adventure day - SUP lessons
Monday 30 Minutes Resistance/ Mobility 10-20 min online cardio class	Tuesday Mobility 40 minutes Walking at PE 3	Wednesday 30 minutes Resistance/ mobility 30 minutes walking at PE 2-3 + HIIT walking	Thursday Rest Mobility	Friday 30 minutes Resistance/ Mobility 30 minutes walking at PE 3	Saturday 45 minute hike adding Stairs/ Hill training	Sunday Rest

Monday	Tuesday	Wednesday	Thursday	Friday	Saturday	Sunday
30 Minutes Resistance/ Mobility Medatative, relaxing walk	Mobility 30 minutes Walking at PE 3 + 1 5 min HIIT walking	30 minutes Resistance/ mobility 30 minutes walking at PE 2-3 + HIIT walking	Rest Mobility	30 Minutes Resistance/ Mobility 30 minutes walking at PE 3	Yin yoga 15-25 min online class 10 minutes of balance work	Adventure day - kayak lessons

Client Example Jacquie - Level One

Client, Jacquie, is another long-time athlete who sought my help because pain, injuries, and mobility issues had completely halted her active lifestyle. She found herself constantly sitting on the couch, reminiscing about her past activities and munching on sugary snacks! While she didn't enjoy mobility exercises, she was willing to try to improve. But, she refused to do any resistance training, weightlifting was out.

Since she didn't want to do resistance training, we focused on 2-3 balance sessions a week, which you now know is another form of bodyweight exercise. :) Additionally, we added indoor cycling since she started her program in the winter, in Canada.

Jacquie didn't need to lose weight, but she did need to dump the sugar and develop a better mindset. Her outlook had become bleak. Despite her many years of being a competitive athlete, she was willing to adopt a beginner's mindset, so we added journaling and meditation to her plan. She needed a new North Star and a calmer brain. Also, she wanted a simple, easy-to-follow plan that was very similar on most days. She didn't want to think about what she needed to do.

She learned to celebrate every bit of progress and growth, regardless of its size. After four months of consistent effort, Jacquie experienced some big breakthroughs. She started re-engaging in activities she loved, like trail running and cycling outside, she hurt less and had much better mobility, and she was willing to tackle a couple of resistance workouts each week.

Jacquie's Month One Training Plan:

Monday	Tuesday	Wednesday	Thursday	Friday	Saturday	Sunday
20 minutes Mobility Balance exercises Focus on low sugar intake 5-10 mediation + journaling	Indoor cycling, easy pace 20-25 minutes 5-10 mediation + journaling	20 minutes Mobility Balance exercises Focus on low sugar intake 5-10 mediation + journaling	Online Yoga class Focus on low sugar intake 5-10 mediation + journaling	20 minutes Mobility Balance exercises Focus on low sugar intake 5-10 mediation + journaling	Adventure day - her choice	Rest day
20 minutes Mobility Balance exercises Focus on low sugar intake 5-10 mediation + journaling	Indoor cycling, easy pace 20-25 minutes 5-10 mediation + journaling	20 minutes Mobility Balance exercises Focus on low sugar intake 5-10 mediation + journaling	Online Yoga class Focus on low sugar intake 5-10 mediation + journaling	20 minutes Mobility Balance exercises Focus on low sugar intake 5-10 mediation + journaling	Indoor cycling with one 3-4 minute HIIT session	Adventure day or rest day

PART 2

Monday	Tuesday	Wednesday	Thursday	Friday	Saturday	Sunday
20 minutes Mobility Balance exercises Focus on low sugar intake 5-10 mediation + journaling	Indoor cycling, easy pace 20-25 minutes 5-10 mediation + journaling	20 minutes Mobility Balance exercises - increased intensity Focus on low sugar intake 5-10 mediation + journaling	Online Yoga class Focus on low sugar intake 5-10 mediation + journaling	20 minutes Mobility Balance exercises - increased intensity Focus on low sugar intake 5-10 mediation + journaling	Adventure day or rest day	Rest
nday 20 minutes Mobility Balance exercises - increased intensity for at least 20 mins Focus on low sugar intake 5-10 mediation + journaling	Tuesday Mobility 30 minutes Walking at PE 3 + 1 5 min HIIT walking	Wednesday 20 minutes Mobility Balance exercises - increased intensity for at least 20 mins Focus on low sugar intake 5-10 mediation + journaling	Online Yoga class Focus on low sugar intake 5-10 mediation + journaling	20 minutes Mobility Balance exercises - increased intensity for at least 20 mins Focus on low sugar intake 5-10 mediation + journaling	Online yoga class	Adventure day

Client Example Susie - Level One

When Susie first approached me to work together, she was possibly below level one! In her late 50s, she had minimal exercise experience, limited to occasional walks and a few aerobic classes decades past. Recently, she had been dealing with knee and hip issues and was truly concerned about her future. She was single with no children and was concerned about what would happen if she couldn't care for herself. Add to this worry about mortality raising its ugly head, and Susie was in a bad place! She was completely unsure about what she would like in her workout plan simply because she'd not done much of anything previously. Unlike most of my clients, she was a blank slate when it came to her preferences, which was a blessing and a curse!

I decided that the best thing we could do was to make month number one fun and exciting, so we made it a test month. Giving Susie a plethora of choices would allow us to see what she liked, didn't like, and could stick to! She tried online classes like; Jazzercise, yoga, Pelatron, Barre, HIIT, and some in-person options like Pilates, yoga, a local hiking club, and a walking group. Through trial and error, she discovered that she really liked the community and accountability aspect of the groups and classes. And she discovered which exercises caused her discomfort (beyond just lactic acid). After her month of trial activities, I had her work with a body alignment coach to strengthen specific areas before diving into resistance training and longer cardio.

By the third month, Susie had developed enough strength and know-how to expand her routine. We incorporated resistance bands to further enhance her strength. Plus, I suggested she dive deeper into hiking because she lived near good trails and really enjoyed the hikes she's been on. By month four, she was almost pain-free, doing things she'd only dreamed of. She could keep up with the group during hikes and even handle tasks like lifting heavy bags of dirt for her garden. She's a movement convert these days and really enjoying everything she had to look forward to!

PART 2

Susie's Month One Training Plan:

Monday	Tuesday	Wednesday	Thursday	Friday	Saturday	Sunday
10 minutes Mobility Online trial class - her choice	10 minutes Mobility Light walk	10 minutes Mobility Online/in person class - her choice	Online Yin Yoga class	10 minutes Mobility	10 minutes Mobility Online/in person class - her choice	Rest day
10 minutes Mobility Online trial class - her choice	10 minutes Mobility Light walk	10 minutes Mobility Online/In person trial class - her choice	Online Yoga or Yin Yoga class	Rest	Rest	Adventure day - Hike
10 minutes Mobility Online trial class - her choice	10 minutes Mobility 20-30 minute walk at PE of 2-3	10 minutes Mobility Online/in person class - her choice	Rest	10 minutes Mobility Online/in person class - her choice	Adventure day or rest day	Rest
10 minutes Mobility Online trial class - her choice	10 minutes Mobility 30 minute walk at PE of 2-3	10 minutes Mobility Online/in person class - her choice	Online Yoga class	10 minutes Mobility Online/in person class - her choice OR 30 minute walk PE of 2-3	Rest	Adventure day

Client Example Lydia - Level Two

Here's a client who began at Level 2. When Lydia joined the group, business, family difficulties, and a lack of prioritizing her health had slowed her down, and her goal was to get in shape and start really enjoying her life. She had always enjoyed activities like pickleball, hiking, golf, and swimming but had been leading a relatively sedentary lifestyle for several years. Even with a solid fitness foundation, her inactivity took a toll on her body. She joined the 12-week Accelerator Program and was rocking it—resistance training three times a week, cardio sessions, mobility, and she quit smoking!

Unfortunately, Lydia started experiencing significant shoulder pain that forced her to come to a halt, which was disheartening, but she wasn't ready to give up! We put her Accelerator Program on hold, and she started working with a physical therapist who had the solution to several body issues she was experiencing. Her shoulder was impacting her entire body. Once her alignment was back, she was back in the Accelerator with renewed enthusiasm. She successfully completed the remaining 12 weeks, plus an additional 24 weeks of the program, Rock Star material!

Throughout her journey, Lydia not only lost inches but also gained muscle definition. Her dedication and effort have been remarkable. Moreover, she now has exciting future adventures to anticipate because she knows she is capable of doing almost anything.

Since Lydia was starting at Level 2, you might notice that her training plan was more extensive than the previous plans. We added more training days plus a lot of mobility to make sure her joints were ready for whatever she did. If you're starting at Level 2, don't feel like you have to start with the same level of activity or intensity. I can't stress enough that your plan is unique to you, and as you go forward, you'll find your optimum exercise plan.

Lydia's Month One Training Plan:

Monday	Tuesday	Wednesday	Thursday	Friday	Saturday	Sunday
10 minutes Mobility Weight Training - upper body	10 minutes Mobility Walk, hike or bike 30 minutes	10 minutes Mobility Weight Training - lower body	10 minutes Mobility Walk, hike or bike 30 minutes and wrap with a 5 min HIIT	10 minutes Mobility Weight Training - full body	10 minutes Mobility or Yoga class Plus - Adventure day	Rest day
Monday	Tuesday	Wednesday	Thursday	Friday	Saturday	Sunday
10 minutes Mobility Training - upper body	10 minutes Mobility Walk, hike or bike 30 - 40 minutes	10 minutes Mobility Weight Training - lower body	10 minutes Mobility Walk, hike or bike 30 minutes and wrap with a 5 min HIIT	10 minutes Mobility Weight Training - full body	10 minutes Mobility or Yoga class Plus - Adventure day	Rest
Monday	Tuesday	Wednesday	Thursday	Friday	Saturday	Sunday
10 minutes Mobility Training - upper body	10 minutes Mobility Walk, hike or bike 30 - 50 minutes	10 minutes Mobility Weight Training - lower body	10 minutes Mobility Walk, hike or bike 30 minutes and wrap with a 5 min HIIT	10 minutes Mobility Weight Training - full body	10 minutes Mobility or Yoga class Plus - Adventure day	Rest
Monday	Tuesday	Wednesday	Thursday	Friday	Saturday	Sunday
10 minutes Mobility Training - upper body	10 minutes Mobility Walk, hike or bike 30 - 40 minutes	10 minutes Mobility Weight Training - lower body	10 minutes Mobility Walk, hike or bike 30 minutes and wrap with a 5 min HIIT	10 minutes Mobility Weight Training - full body	10 minutes Mobility or Yoga class Plus - Adventure day	Rest

Client Example Dana - Level Two

Another Level 2 client, Dana, had been a part of the Fit is Freedom Community for about a year. During one of our group calls, she participated in a Future Self meditation, where we focus on connecting with the woman we want to be; six months, a year, or even further in the future. Through this exercise, Dana identified she wanted more out of her fitness; she wanted to feel really good in her own skin and be able to smile genuinely when she caught her reflection in a passing mirror. Inspired and wanting so much more, she joined our 12 week accelerator program, which she later extended for an additional 12 weeks.

Throughout the program, her significant achievement wasn't weight loss, which she went into the program thinking was her goal. Instead, she gained muscle and lost several inches in her stomach and hips. Excited by the woman in the mirror, she purchased an entirely new wardrobe, so now she has a double smile when she catches her reflection! Today, she genuinely feels good in her own skin.

Dana's program was straightforward. She engaged in resistance training three days a week, followed by various forms of cardio. Since she enjoys dance activities, one of her resistance days is a Jazzercise class incorporating weights. Despite nasty cold weather and a lot of travel, she stayed 100% consistent with her program, and her efforts show!

PART 2

Dana's Month One Training Plan:

Monday	Tuesday	Wednesday	Thursday	Friday	Saturday	Sunday
10 minutes Mobility Weight Training - full body	Mat Pilates	10 minutes Mobility Weight Training - full body	10 minutes Mobility Walk, hike or bike 30 minutes and wrap with a 5 min HIIT	10 minutes Mobility Jazzercise w/weights	Adventure day or Rest day	Rest day
10 minutes Mobility Weight Training - full body	10 minutes Mobility 30 minute cardio of choice	10 minutes Mobility Weight Training - full body	10 minutes Mobility 30 minute cardio of choice wrap with a 5 min HIIT	10 minutes Mobility Jazzercise w/weights	10 minutes Mobility or Yoga class Plus - Adventure day or Rest day	Rest
10 minutes Mobility Weight Training - full body	10 minutes Mobility 30 minute cardio of choice or day off	10 minutes Mobility Weight Training - full body	10 minutes Mobility Walk, hike or bike 30 minutes and wrap with a 5 min HIIT	10 minutes Mobility Jazzercise w/weights or day off	10 minutes Mobility or Yoga class Plus - Adventure day	Rest
10 minutes Mobility Weight Training - full body	10 minutes Mobility Walk, hike or bike 30 minutes and wrap with a 5 min HIIT	10 minutes Mobility Weight Training - full body	10 minutes Mobility Walk, hike or bike 30 minutes and wrap with a 5 min HIIT	10 minutes Mobility Weight Training - full body or Jazzercise w/weights or day off	Rest or Adventure day	Rest

Client Example Jackie - Level 3

A Level 3 client, Jackie, had a strong fitness foundation from our years of working together. She was vibrant, felt great, slept great, and was happy with her size. However, after undergoing an unexpected surgery, her recovery took almost 10 weeks longer than expected. During this time, she started losing muscle, plus her good outlook on life! When you're used to being active, your body and brain don't appreciate the downtime.

It was challenging for her to stay positive and believe this slump would end. Once she received approval from her doctor, we started her fitness recovery with a slow and gentle approach. We began with three days of light resistance training, adding stairs one day a week (since she enjoyed them) and two long walks. One of the walks included 10-20 minutes of high-intensity training, while the other was as long as she desired, serving as a way to clear her mind. Additionally, we addressed her plummeting mood by incorporating short meditations, around five minutes or less, and five minutes of journaling. Jackie discovered a love for journaling and extended her sessions to 15 minutes and then even more. Combining mindset work into her recovery, Jackie made remarkable progress. By month four post-surgery, she had surpassed her previous fitness level.

Jackie's Month One Training Plan:

Monday	Tuesday	Wednesday	Thursday	Friday	Saturday	Sunday
Meditation & Journaling 20 minutes Mobility Weight Training - full body with bands	Meditation & Journaling Easy walk & Stair workout	Meditation & Journaling 20 minutes Mobility Weight Training - full body with bands	Meditation & Journaling 10 minutes Mobility Walk or hike 30 minutes+ and wrap with a 10 min HIIT	Meditation & Journaling 20 minutes Mobility Weight Training - full body with bands	Meditation & Journaling Adventure day or Rest day	Adventure day or Rest day
Monday	Tuesday	Wednesday	Thursday	Friday	Saturday	Sunday
Meditation & Journaling 20 minutes Mobility Weight Training - full body with bands	Meditation & Journaling Easy walk & Stair workout	Meditation & Journaling 20 minutes Mobility Weight Training - full body with bands	Meditation & Journaling 10 minutes Mobility Walk or hike 30 minutes+ and wrap with a 10 min HIIT	Meditation & Journaling 20 minutes Mobility Weight Training - full body with bands	Meditation & Journaling Yoga class Plus - Adventure day or Rest day	Rest

Monday	Tuesday	Wednesday	Thursday	Friday	Saturday	Sunday
Meditation & Journaling 20 minutes Mobility Weight Training - full body with bands	Meditation & Journaling Easy walk & Stair workout	Meditation & Journaling 20 minutes Mobility Weight Training - full body with bands	Meditation & Journaling 10 minutes Mobility Walk or hike 30 minutes+ and wrap with a 10 min HIIT	Meditation & Journaling 20 minutes Mobility Weight Training - full body with bands	Meditation & Journaling Plus - Adventure day	Rest
Monday	Tuesday	Wednesday	Thursday	Friday	Saturday	Sunday
Meditation & Journaling 10 minutes Mobility Weight Training - full body with light hand weights	Meditation & Journaling Easy walk & Stair workout	Meditation & Journaling 10 minutes Mobility Weight Training - full body with light hand weights	Meditation & Journaling 10 minutes Mobility Walk or hike 30 minutes+ and wrap with a 10 min HIIT	Meditation & Journaling 10 minutes Mobility Weight Training - full body with light hand weights	Meditation & Journaling Rest or Adventure day	Rest

Your Turn - Sample Plan Level One:

Now that you've seen some real-life examples, it's your turn! Let's pretend that you have 40 minutes a day, four days a week maximum, to exercise. You have some joint pain, but your doctor has given you the green light to exercise and suggests resistance training is very important! Your goals are: to lose weight, gain muscle, increase your energy, and be able to keep up with your friends on a hike. You do not have access to a gym or classes except online, but you do live near a park or a neighborhood where you can walk.

Given your limited time options, you opt for an online mobility program and resistance band training. You enjoy walking, but in the past, you've found that you are more of a stroller than a power walker. You decide to up your walking effort and add in little walking HIIT sessions, and since you're willing to sweat more these days, you even throw in some stair/hill training. Your month one plan could look something like this

Level One - Month One Example

Week One: (Theme - start slow)

- Mobility - 10 minutes a day, 4 days a week
- Resistance - 20 minutes a day, 2-3 days a week
- Cardio: walking - 20 minutes a day, 3 days a week at a perceived effort (PE) of 2 to 3 day
- Cardio: walking - 25 minutes at perceived effort (PE) of 2 to 3 day plus 5 minute 1 HIIT

Week Two: (Theme - build)

- Mobility- 10 minutes a day, 4 days a week
- Resistance - continue with 20 minutes a day, 4 days a week, using FitForever.com

- Cardio: walking - 20 minutes a day, 2 days a week at a perceived effort (PE) of 2 to 3 days with two days adding in 2 HIIT sessions of 5 minutes each.
- Cardio: online, low impact 10-20 minute cardio class

Week Three: (Theme - build)

- Mobility - 10 minutes a day, 4 days a week
- Resistance - continue with 20 minutes a day, 4 days a week, using FitForever.com
- Cardio 1: walking - 20 minutes a day, 2 days a week at a perceived effort (PE) of 3 after you warm up and adding 1 HIIT session at the end of 5 minutes.
- Cardio 2: two online, low impact 20 minutes cardio classes
- Cardio 3: Stairs/Hill training. Find somewhere you can walk and include stairs or hills for 25 minutes. Mix flat with elevation. If you live somewhere hilly, just go up a hill part way, return slowly and carefully back to the bottom, and then walk flat for 3-5 minutes. If you live somewhere flat, get creative. You can use a parking garage or the side of a local overpass. Start looking now for potential places to do light hill work. If the weather is inclement, use indoor steps either in your house if possible. REMEMBER - if you have any balance issues use handrails or walking poles.

Week Four: (theme - rest and rejuvenate)

- Mobility - 10 minutes a day, 5 days a week
- Resistance - continue with 20 minutes a day, 3 days a week
- Cardio: walking - 20 minutes a day, 2 days a week at a perceived effort (PE) of 2-3 after you warm up.
- Balance & Rest - enjoy two 15-minute Yin Yoga workouts from an online video and then do 5 minutes of balance work, remembering to have an accessible handhold and

simple moves like; one foot in front, behind, and to the side.

As you design this plan, it will look something like this:

Monday	Tuesday	Wednesday	Thursday	Friday	Saturday	Sunday
20 Minutes Resistance/ mobility	20 minutes Walking at PE2-3	20 minutes Resistance/ mobility 20 minutes walking at PE 2-3	Rest day	20 minutes Resistance/ Mobility 20 minutes walking at PE 2-3	25 minutes walking at PE 2-3 15 minute HIIT session	Rest day
Monday 20 Minutes Resistance/ Mobility 10-20 min online cardio class	Tuesday 20 minutes Resistance/ Mobility 20 minutes Walking at PE2-3	Wednesday 20 minutes Resistance/ Mobility 20 minutes Walking at PE2-3 include 1 5min HIIT session	Thursday Rest	Friday 20 minutes Resistance/ Mobility 20 minutes walking at PE 2-3	Saturday 30 minutes walking at PE 2-3 15 minute HIIT session	Sunday Rest

Monday	Tuesday	Wednesday	Thursday	Friday	Saturday	Sunday
20 Minutes Resistance/Mobility 10-20 min online cardio class	20 Minutes Resistance/Mobility	20 Minutes Resistance/Mobility 20 minutes walking at (PE) of 3 after warm up and adding 1 HIIT session the last 5 minutes	Rest	20 Minutes Resistance/Mobility 20 minutes walking at (PE) of 3 after warm up and adding 1 HIIT session the last 5 minutes	25 minutes walking plus Stairs/Hill training	Rest
Monday	Tuesday	Wednesday	Thursday	Friday	Saturday	Sunday
20 Minutes Resistance/Mobility 20 minutes Walking at PE2-3	20 Minutes Resistance/Mobility	20 Minutes Resistance/Mobility 20 minutes Walking at PE2-3	Rest	20 Minutes Resistance/Mobility Yin yoga 15 min online class plus short balance work	Yin yoga 15 min online class 5 minutes of balance work	Adventure day - what will you do?

Your turn. Remember, start slow and small. Plan for plenty of fun throughout the month. Most importantly, you do not need to be perfect with your plan. If you hit 80-90% of your workouts, you are on the path to everything you desire! Take your time and have fun with this. You will find an editable monthly calendar in your Freedom Journal or use the outline below.

_____

_____

PART 2

Monday	Tuesday	Wednes- day	Thursday	Friday	Saturday	Sunday
Monday	Tuesday	Wednes- day	Thursday	Friday	Saturday	Sunday
Monday	Tuesday	Wednes- day	Thursday	Friday	Saturday	Sunday
Monday	Tuesday	Wednes- day	Thursday	Friday	Saturday	Sunday
Monday	Tuesday	Wednes- day	Thursday	Friday	Saturday	Sunday

Bottom Line

Create your plan, and try it out. Make changes as needed and then reassess. This is not a perfect science, this is life. Messy, fun, changeable, and unpredictable life. Always remember, progress not perfection. Keep moving forward one small step at a time and enjoy the journey! As you get better at creating your plan, it will become easier and quicker!

In the next chapter, you'll find a series of quick wins and client suggestions to help bring even more life and ideas to your plan!

CHAPTER 7.5
STARTING AND STAYING CONSISTENT

By now, I'm sure you've come to believe that fitness is physical and mental! In order to set ourselves to win any time we start something new, we need to make it easy. The more support and clarity we have, the higher our success rate. In this chapter, we start with several mindset tips, move on to important fitness tricks and wrap up with plenty of real-life wisdom from the Fit is Freedom community!

You are the Priority

Let's talk about priorities. We prioritize what matters most to us. Have you made your health and wellness your priority? Great. When you do, you have just said that you are going to be here for your family because you're taking care of yourself. When you are willing to prioritize your fitness, you are saying that you're ready for more. You're ready for a life that gives you freedom and fun. You must be the priority.

What time commitment will you prioritize? Commit to what is realistic, and then stick to it. This is your time. Commit. Make your plan. Take action. You are the priority in that time you have given to yourself!

Think of this as an Experiment

In my Fit is Freedom group, we do monthly experiments. Experiments are when we focus on one particular area for 30 days. We might concentrate on balance, sugar freedom, sleep, fitness tracking, etc. These months are called an Experiment for a reason. When we call it an experiment, it arouses curiosity and lessens the rules. When we ask questions like what do I like about this, what about this works, what don't I like, how do I feel, the pressure is off, and we get curious. A curious mind is open to new possibilities.

When you use hard and fast rules - do this, don't do that, all the 'shoulds' come up. If we don't get something exactly correct, we stop because we are not doing it 'right.' When you make it an experiment, you can observe what works, what doesn't work, what you like, and what you quite frankly hate. You're then armed with information and knowledge to move forward, empowered. You won't quit yet again because you didn't fit into someone else's idea of what you should or shouldn't do!

Use Open Loops

When you're having trouble finishing what you start, whether it's repetitions while you're strength training, doing HIIT intervals, or finishing your mobility work - use open loops.

An open loop is when your brain sees unfinished business, and our brains don't like open loops. Suppose you decide to do five fast-slow intervals at the end of your walk. Count them down, 5-4-3-2-1, not up. When you count down, 5-4-3, typically, you won't quit at 3. If you're counting up, you just might start negotiating with yourself at number 3...*I can stop now and do more on Thursday*...it won't happen on Thursday!

HIIT reimagined

Suggestions on how to do (HIIT) High Intensity Interval Training can be intimidating. I prefer to keep it very simple; a 1 to 2 or 1 to 3 ratio works just fine for getting started. For example, let's say that you're walking for your cardio. Occasionally, at the end of the walk, commit to a number of interval sets. All these sets entail is walking fast (perceived effort 4-5) for 30 seconds, then walking slow (perceived effort 1-2) for 60 seconds, the 1 to 2 ratio. Continue this flow for your predetermined number of sets. If you can't do 30 seconds, go hard for 10 seconds, and slow for 30 seconds, a 1 to 3 ratio. Do what works for you. Make it easy on yourself while still getting your heart rate up, bring it back down, and then increase it again.

Have an MDM Plan (Minimum Daily Movement)

We all have those days, the ones where everything goes sideways and your well laid plans fall apart. One day like this won't stop your forward progress, but two or more, and you need to have an MDM to fall back on. An MDM is a very simple movement plan based on the idea that a body in motion stays in motion. You want your MDM to be so quick and easy that there's simply no way you can say; I don't have time, this is too much today, I'm too tired.

MDMs will vary for everyone. In the Fit is Freedom community, one of the go-to MDMs is what we call Nitros. Based on Dr. Zack Bush's Nitric Workout, it's 4 simple moves that take less than 10 minutes that pack a health punch. You can find a copy of this video at www.FitisFreedom.com/bonuses. Typically, 2-3 nitros in a day is a perfect MDM plan.

Your MDM might be a 10-minute walk and 5 minutes of yoga. It varies for everyone, but the bottom line is to keep an MDM that you can do almost anywhere, anytime you are missing a scheduled workout. Keep moving. Once you develop the habit of consistent movement, you'll find that staying on track and getting back on track is a breeze.

Balance is Strength

If you find yourself fighting the idea of resistance training, start with balance work. Balance is typically not the first thing we think of when we think of exercise. Still, it is the secret ingredient in almost everything we do! From taking a leisurely hike, rising from a cozy chair without using our arms, to standing up on a standup paddleboard - it's all about balance. Having strong muscles and practicing steadiness makes balance a breeze.

Balance training exercises strengthen the muscles that keep us upright, especially our legs and core. These exercises boost our stability and act as our personal bodyguards preventing falls.

Want to step it up? Use equipment like a Bosu half-circle stability ball or a balance board, or even a soft foam pad. Practice where you can easily catch yourself if your balance is off one day. The back of a solid chair, a counter, or a tabletop. Keep them in arm's reach.

Track Perceived Effort

My favorite way to track how hard a client is working is by using Perceived Effort. It's easy to track with zero apps or devices and teaches you to become more in tune with your body. Consider when you're walking and carrying on a conversation with a friend. At a perceived effort of 1, your conversation would be so easy that no one would notice that you're exerting any effort – think of a casual stroll with a friend.

At a perceived effort of 2, you're working a little harder, but it's still not much of anything. As you reach a perceived effort of 3, you can carry on a conversation, but if someone was talking to you on the phone, they could tell you were exercising, but you could still carry on a conversation. At a 4, you're definitely feeling the effect of what you are doing! And, at a perceived effort of 5, you're going full out. A conversation is almost impossible, if at all. You can only focus on what you're doing. You may have to work with this a few times, but as you do, it quickly becomes intuitive. Going forward, you'll automatically consider your perceived effort and adjust your fitness effect to fit your workout.

Track Your Workouts and Your Achievements

When you track your workouts, you can look back and see where you've come from and how you've improved! Personally, I like to track time, distance, and perceived effort to see how my fitness is increasing. Let's say it takes you 22 minutes to do a mile at a perceived effort of 3-4. Write it down and then 3-4 weeks later, track it again. You might see that now it's taking you 21 minutes to finish that mile, and your perceived effort is a solid 3. #WIN!

Have Rest Days and Pivot When Needed

Rest also matters. It matters when you build muscle (muscle is built while you rest, not while you lift). It matters when you start feeling a touch of burn. It really matters when something begins to feel uncomfortable in a joint, DON'T keep pushing. Rest is recovery. My typical week includes 1-2 rest days. If I've been pushing hard, I may have 3 or more rest days. On rest days, I almost always do a few minutes of mobility. Or a session of Yin Yoga. Something that will keep my body moving gently, not pushing hard. Always schedule rest days into your schedule.

The need to pivot happens! There will be days when life happens and your schedule doesn't go according to plan, that's when it is time to give yourself a little grace and do a pivot!

Didn't make it to the gym? Do a longer walk than usual

Unexpected company? Change your rest day and enjoy your company.

Poor night's sleep stopped you from a workout? Focus on mobility and balance for the day, and give yourself a rest.

Life happens. Plan for the best, and then work with what you have!

Fit is Freedom Friend - Isabella

When we first started working together, Isabella did one thing and one thing only. She went for a one-hour walk every day. As perceived effort went, she was at a 2, tops. She'd been doing her walks since her doctor told her two years before that she was headed for a heart attack and needed to start walking. But nothing was happening. She still had high blood pressure, she was still on medication, her weight was the same, her sleep was poor, and her moods were dark.

She was referred to me by one of my clients. When we first talked, she told me what she'd been doing. I suggested a few small changes, and she said no, that wasn't what her doctor had suggested. Okay. I wasn't going against what her doctor said, so it looked like I couldn't help her myself. I gave her a list of coaches and professionals that I referred people to and wished her the best.

About a month later, I was surprised to see her name on my call calendar!

When we got on her call, it turned out she had gone back to her doctor and was told that "just walking wasn't making a difference. She needed to do something else." Perfect. I knew she had the drive and the time because, for two years, she had walked almost every day. That's commitment.

So we took that one hour a day and built out a new plan. Her plan included some walking because we loved it, but she picked up the pace and only went for about 20 to 40 minutes a day. We added mobility 4 days a week and resistance training from Fit Forever 4 times a week. We also added a little HIIT time (once a week) and rest in the form of restorative yoga. When her plan was done, she was spending a little less time each week, but she was going to be much more effective!

Then, we added the no-fun for her portion. She started working on her sugar addiction. She had been in total denial about her nutrition for many years. Less sugar, more vegetables, better carbs, more protein, and good fats. A very basic eating plan but one that was quite different than what she's been doing.

She leaned in on accountability with the Fit is Freedom community and me. We'll talk more about how to use the right type of accountability in Chapter 10, but for now, just know we all had her back!

It took a year (which sounds like a long time unless you've wanted to change for years!). But, over that year, her life completely transformed. She went from frequently sad to happy, genuinely happy. She made friends in the community, and they made plans together. She changed jobs, lost weight (about 25 pounds), got off her medication, and is planning to walk the Camino de Santiago in 2024.

I am so grateful she returned after that first call, and she frequently tells me how grateful she is too. Godspeed to you on the Camino, my friend!

Although your dream may not be walking the Camino de Santiago… start thinking about what your might be…

Follow Your North Star To Keep Moving Forward

Dream time! Grab your Freedom Journal and start writing. In your wildest dreams, what do you want the next few months to bring? What do you want to accomplish that will light you up? This is not an exercise about potentially losing weight or fitting into that certain pair of pants. Forget those for a moment and focus on what excites you. I promise weight will come off as you start moving more. What matters most is how you are feeling and what you can do! Go back to Chapter 4 and revisit your North Star. What does being fit and free mean to you?

Your fitness goals can be anything that truly matters to you. The more life-changing, the better.

- Amy is training for her grandkids, they love hiking, camping, and kayaking, and she is excitedly planning to be there every step of the way.

- Susie had a health scare two years ago and realized that if she didn't change her habits ASAP, her health (and thus her life) was heading downhill, fast, and that wasn't how she wanted to live. Today her health issues are behind her, she's going places she never thought would be possible, and she has a new romance in her life.

- Nina broke her ankle and was incapacitated for 6 months. After getting the all-clear from her doctor, she stepped up her walking and added yoga and mobility work to her plan because all the months of no movement had her hurting in places that had never been a problem before. Today she is pain-free, she's dropped the 25 pounds she gained during recovery, and she leads bike rides and hikes in her community!

- Kris had a really big dream that deep down she never believed would happen…hiking the entire Pacific Rim Trail! Guess what? She's doing it this year. It's been her secret dream for decades. She followed her training plan, found two women to hike with, and she's heading out this summer. The power of dreams.

PART 2

Wisdom From The Fit is Freedom Community

I asked one of our Accountability Text Groups to share what holds them back from creating a weekly workout plan and what encourages them to do it, so straight from these amazing women's words:

- "I am a very time-conscious person, so making a plan comes easy to me, but it has to be fun and something I enjoy!" - Viviann

- "What was stopping me, I think, was that subconsciously I was afraid that if I wrote it down, if I made it 'real', then I'd reproach myself if I didn't do what I said I would do. I would make vague plans in my head, but there's no evidence (or even clear memory) of what those vague plans were. So writing my plan down, putting it somewhere visible, and checking things off as I complete them, has been a revelation for me" - Lee

- "Writing it down is helpful. I schedule all my meetings at work, time with family, tasks to accomplish, it only makes sense to put aside time to plan my workout, and I finally find I get it done." - Deidre

- "What kept me from writing down my weekly schedule? Plain and simple, it wasn't in my routines and habits. Not that I'm forming a new version of myself: I need to formally commit to a plan and schedule my fitness. I won't say there isn't an underlying trepidation that I won't accomplish what's on the schedule and thus not measure up to being who I want to be at the end of this journey 📱♀ …And really, I'd still like to be that person that doesn't have to bother with details—just magically fit and slim. Honestly, it aggravates me sometimes. But I'm getting better every week!" - Sarah

- "I've always felt if I write it down, then I'm locked into that, and we all know life is full of the unexpected. To-

day is a prime example, everything went sideways, and I didn't get to the gym. Before Fit is Freedom and working with Kelly, I would have been, "well crap, I've blown the workout today before the day even started." Instead, I've learned to think differently. Maybe I can get a cardio workout from a video and do my Nitros throughout the day. The day isn't lost like I would have thought at one time. I just change gears instead of cussing myself now."
- Pam

> *"Having a schedule and then allowing myself to pivot and pick something else off my weekly workout changes everything"* - Everyone

You now have everything you need to succeed.

Having a written plan and quick wins that will keep you on track helps to remove the need for motivation or, worse, trying to depend on willpower. Willpower isn't sustainable. It runs out fast, especially when we lean on it again and again. Conversely, I've noticed that the more consistent we are, the more willpower we have. Experiments have shown it's not the type of movement you do, but simply that you picked a movement plan and stuck to it will raise willpower and self-control significantly!

Sometimes clients will say to me something like: "I'm just not as motivated [or driven] as you are." The reality is I'm not always motivated. There are days I'd rather not worry about my workouts and days I feel like I can't squeeze another thing in.

This is when the power of habits kicks in.

In our next chapter, we'll look at any habits that may have halted your progress in the past and how to change them forever by simply learning the magic of **Habit Shifting.** Changing habits can be tough, but learning how to implement simple habits shifts makes it a breeze.

CHAPTER 8
FORGET CHANGING HABITS: SIMPLY SHIFT THEM!

"Einstein said, "The measure of intelligence is the ability to change." I would add to that; the ability to change again and again and again until we get it right." - Kelly

Habits. Such a charged word! And something I'd rather not bring up, but any change worth doing almost always involves changing a habit or five. And as anyone who has tried to change lifelong habits knows, it can be tough! Like the proverbial New Year's Resolutions, we might approach our new fitness plan with ridged goals and hard timelines.

"I'm going to lose 20 pounds in two months."

"I'm going to workout 6 days a week."

"I'm quitting sugar for good."

When we lean on willpower, if life gets busy, willpower gives out (usually about week three). Before we know it, we're back to the "next week, next month, this summer, then I'll get serious about my fitness plan" mantra.

Successful women are used to succeeding. That's why failing at fitness consistency hurts so much. It feels like a dog chasing its tail, circling and circling until it hits the ground. Never quite getting there. After twenty-plus years of working with all these strong, amazing, successful women who at one time struggled to stay consistent with their fitness, I've come to believe we approach change wrongly.

Instead of stomping in with our all-or-nothing Superwoman cape on, ready to change everything, what if we start small and keep shifting what isn't working until it's exactly what we want?

Suzan was recently retired, and after years of following her bosses' schedule, she wasn't interested in a hard and fast fitness plan. It became a bit of an inside joke. I would ask her if she had outlined her fitness plan for the week, and she would say: "Nope, I don't need a plan. I want to be able to do what feels good for me each day." I'd smile, check in with her and note that she was hitting maybe 20% of her fitness plan we'd created together. Actually, her plan was gathering dust. And she was gathering a little extra around the waist. We would meet each week, and I'd ask her if she'd been tracking her food or her workouts (which she said she wanted to do), and she would get a petulant look on her face and say, "I'm doing something most days." But she wasn't. And, since she wasn't getting results, I didn't like taking her money.

We were at an impasse.

As the weeks went by, she became less motivated, I was frustrated, and when she said, "Maybe this isn't for me, maybe my fitness is as good as it's ever going to get," we decided to go our separate ways.

Fortunately or unfortunately, I have a stubborn streak. I knew in my heart that with just a few small habits shifts, her life and her future would change completely. That's why two days later, we were on a call together, yet again. I'd come up with this crazy, habit-shifting-and-stacking-fitness-plan-that-didn't-look-like-a-plan at all idea. (Habit-stacking is when you tie a habit you desire to a current habit that you have set in stone; the good ones like brushing your teeth and going to sleep at the right time). My ulterior motive behind her new non-plan was to get her past seeing only hard effort and instead to see that an easy path to freedom was just around the corner.

I'll tell you the rest of Susan's story in a minute, but first, let's talk about why changing habits is so problematic.

First, most of us have had our habits for a very long time. In fact, I'm willing to bet that the majority of our habits were learned early, which means those habits belonged not just to us but to our parents too. Habits are sticky and a little like an old friend. When we think we need to get rid of a habit, heels dig in, and that inner little kid feeling of "I don't want to change" or "No fun food forever? Forget it!" pops up. Or even worse, we get that sick feeling in the pit of our stomach that leads us to think… "I've tried to change so many times, but it never works, so why do I even want to try again?"

This is why I created my Habit Shifting Method. What if instead of forcing change, we slipped up on it, lightly changing this and shifting that and then pausing to see how it feels? And then take the next step and the one after that until one day you look backward and see how these small steps have taken you to the top of the mountain!

Before we go over my Habit Shifting Method, let's take a quick look at the very conventional and effective habit stacking. Habit stacking is when you anchor a new habit to an existing one. The pros of habit stacking are that you already have a habit in place, you're just adding to it. The cons of habit stacking is it can be a little cumbersome, needing to remember when you are doing this one action, you need to be doing the other action also.

Examples could be brushing your teeth becomes brushing teeth and hip mobility moves to get the day started. Or doing squats while the coffee brews or countertop push-ups as food is warming in the microwave.

Personally, I find habit stacking a little much. I might plan to "stack some habits," but I get busy and forget. Or, the flipside comes up when you want to quit a current habit; what do you tie your habit stacking to? Let me be really clear, the habit stacking method works, but I'm always looking for the easy path. When it comes to habit shifting over habit stacking, I prefer shifting because I forget to stack habits, even when I make a plan to stack!

Suppose you'd like to learn more about habits. In that case, two books I'd suggest are *The Power of Habit* by Charles Duhigg, a fascinating immersion into the science of habits that's a fun read. And *Atomic Habits* by James Clear is the go-to book for all things habit stacking, another fascinating book on habits and how they evolve and are created.

Habits make our lives easier. They remove the need to make conscience decisions or focus on mundane processes. Habits save us time and effort. They aren't bad. We need to be aware of the ones that don't serve us and then gently and with focused attention start shifting them.

One Small Habit Shift at a Time.

Our brain follows a habitual pattern known as the habit loop whenever we engage in a repeated response. This loop consists of several stages, commencing with a trigger that prompts a craving, followed by an action, and ultimately culminating in a reward. Triggers can manifest in various forms, including emotions, specific locations or times, other individuals, visuals, and more. They induce a craving within us for something we may not have thought much about just moments prior, such as sugar, wine, ice cream, or a particular TV show. Suddenly, we find ourselves consumed by the desire to have it. Subsequently, we respond by taking action, firmly convinced that it will improve our situation or fulfill our needs (establishing a routine). Finally, the reward phase ensues as we yield to our cravings in that particular moment.

When it comes to an unwanted or undesirable habit, there is an underlying element that will stop us from changing every time: The emotional side of the shame, disgust, feelings of failing yet again, and the physical discomfort that comes from eating the bag of candy, hitting the chocolate, having the extra wine. In my book, this is potentially the worse step in this loop. Because when we are not happy with ourselves and our actions, it's easy to go further down the black hole of unwanted habits.

It's important to stop this spiral before it begins.

My job is to get you from your fitness WHY to a sustainable, consistent plan as quickly as I can and then help you refocus on your fitness lifestyle again and again for the rest of your life. When "bad" habits slow us down, or not having the right habit in place holds us back, our forward momentum slows. To get moving and keep you moving, I suggest my Habit Shifting Method. Use this easy method to create a new habit or alter a current one. Habit shifting starts with awareness and then follows a path of small repeatable steps. Like a flowing stream or path in the woods, follow the easiest flow for you. Begin with judgment-free awareness and curiosity.

Applying the Habit Shifting Method

Now that you have been introduced to the powerful world of habit-sifting, it is time to guide you on how to do it in your own life.

Step 1. How much does this new habit matter to you? Creating a new habit is slightly different than getting rid of an unwanted habit. Think about the new habit you want. No judgment, just think about how it would matter to you. That's a key point, does it matter to you? Like Suzan in our earlier example, even though she said she wanted a fitness plan, she had no desire to add something that looked like more work or what she left at her old job. The structure made her feel like she'd traded one boss for another. Not what she wanted. Once you know, this is something that you truly want, that can make a desired change in your life, next is awareness.

Step 2. Awareness is key. Take a couple of days and pay attention to your current schedule; when you're busy, when you're most motivated (usually in the morning but not everyone), when you find yourself wasting time and how much time you waste, when you spend time doing things you don't enjoy or that don't make a difference in your life. Pay attention to how much you watch TV, mess around on social media, etc. Don't make any changes, only get curious.

We go through our days on autopilot. Each action was finetuned over years of repetition. As if by route, the alarm leads to the coffee leads to the shower leads to…this is called automaticity, and it allows us to deal with everyday life so we aren't overwhelmed. This is a good thing, except when we want to add or change a habit. We need to rewire the automation.

I recently hired a Spanish teacher. We meet in the afternoons via Zoom. It's been a bit of a struggle for me. My work days can be intense, with many tasks and switching jobs as I go through the day. I found that going from client calls, writing, planning, and team meetings and then straight into Spanish, my concentration wasn't good. I felt like a bad teenager sneaking glimpses at the clock on my phone, is class over yet?!?

But I was not a teenager, and this was something I wanted to do. Why was I so tired and distracted, and what could I do about it? Two things stood out after a few days of paying attention. One was that I was out of calories at 3:30 or 4:00, when the classes typically began. My brain needed fuel! The second thing was I needed a "bridge" between my normal work day and jumping into something completely new and different. Now, about fifteen minutes before my class, I either stop and do a quick meditation or use my Lumosity App to stimulate my brain differently. Spanish is still hard, but I'm no longer peeking at the clock!

Step 3. Get very, very curious. Ask yourself better questions and focus on where you can take different actions. Grab your freedom journal and answer the following questions:

- If what I've been doing isn't working, what if I tried XYZ?
- If I mastered my fitness consistency, what would I be doing differently?
- What new activities or actions would I take if I focused on my fitness North Star?

The goal of this step is not to overwhelm or chastise yourself but to just ask questions that give you better answers. Focusing on what's not working dulls our creativity, and getting curious stimulates it.

Step 4. Make a plan. In theory, you already made your fitness plan when you finished the last chapter…but stretch out a straightforward plan if you're still thinking instead of acting. If you're unsure what to do, list 2-5 actions that you can try and test for round one.

Step 5. Take action. Then, of course, quit thinking and start doing. Take imperfect action and keep going daily.

Step 6. Use all your senses. Get visual, auditory, and kinesthetic! Feel how you want to feel. We learn best when we dive deep and immerse ourselves in a new experience. Get creative and use all your senses.

Step 7. Test and Track your ability to follow your plan without judgment. Simply track how well you are doing, how often you follow your plan, and where you fall off and why. And always have zero judgment.

Step 8. No judgment. Awareness without judgment is critical here. If you start judging yourself, expecting perfection, and feeling like you lack progress, you'll quit and fall into the trap of believing you're just not cut out for this…that you might as well throw in the towel.

Step 9. Time. Be willing for this to take time, but don't waiver from your desired outcome. Understand that habit shifting can take time. You've had plenty of time to create these habits! Be gentle and keep bringing yourself back on track.

Step 10. Rinse and repeat as you add new habits and changes you want to embrace. You'll notice that your new habits grow with you.

Fit is Freedom Friend - Suzan. Creating a New Habit (continued)

Let's circle back to what happened when Suzan and I revisited her dislike of having a weekly planning habit.

Two things became apparent; first, I realized that we needed to create a fitness habit for her, it wasn't in her DNA. And second, I realized I was personally being obstinate! Instead of me continuing to insist that Suzan create and follow her weekly fitness plan, we got creative and started habit-shifting and stacking like crazy! We made it a game. Teeth brushing and coffee percolating (whoa, that aged me) became opportunities to tie her mobility moves to something she already did each day. Habit stacking.

Then, we got curious and looked for ways to shift what she was currently doing in her day. She had a much older dog who still wanted to walk every day, albeit a very slow walk which currently was zero exercise for her. She bought a leash belt and wrist weights and started doing resistance training while on the walk, which motivated her to keep going and finish her resistance workout when she got home.

Since cardio was never her favorite, we found other ways she could have camaraderie and break a sweat simultaneously. Pickleball and walking with friends was the answer. As she started tracking her exercise, she noticed that she wasn't doing as much as she thought. She also noticed that she was out of breath quicker than her friends, which she didn't like at all. Instead of feeling bad about her fitness level (remember, no judgment), we added two short weekly HIIT workouts. After using this plan for six weeks, she naturally started creating a structured one. These days she still balks at scheduling her fitness day by day, so she has a system of 'movement units' she created. She even admits that she occasionally makes a structured plan when she knows she'll be traveling or busy.

A big win from Suzan and a great lesson for me! Changing or stopping a habit that you currently have is just slightly different than adding a new habit. Here are a few fine points to be aware of:

Desire, you must have the desire to shift the habit you no longer want, but you don't need to strive for perfection, just improvement. In the Sugar Freedom example below, we look at cutting down on sugar, not stopping consumption forever. It's probably not necessary to cut all sweets out of your life, but if you're overindulging, you make changes. Another powerful way to connect to your desire is to ask yourself; how does this habit stop you from reaching your North Star?

Awareness is the biggest step in removing a habit. Become aware of everything that surrounds this habit. Is it something that is caused by a trigger? Time, emotion, location, person, hunger, and being tired are all triggers that push our buttons and have us act in ways we would rather not. When you are aware of your triggers, you can circumvent the behavior. When you're unaware, you're a reactive mess.

Start small or start big - you have to be the judge. This is something you need to decide on your own. Some people find going "cold turkey" on a habit as best; others like to chop away at it, piece by piece. You'll hear how we do both in the Sugar Freedom example below. Stop sugar completely for 30 days, and then slowly add a few treats or foods we truly love. There's a good reason for this. Suppose you tell yourself that you'll never have sugar or (insert your unhealthy habit here… wine, pasta, staying up too late, too much screentime…). In that case, there will be a revolt in your brain. The little kid inside will cross her arms and chant, "That's not fair."

That inner revolt will stop change, cold.

Come back to awareness and also track your progress. We love to see progress. In our toolbox chapter, we'll dive deeper into tracking. Remember, when your mind can see progress, you'll have better results, so track everything and give your mind visual results. This is why people do so well at the beginning of a diet but then drop off. When you see progress, you move forward. But, when you hit a weight plateau and don't see progress, the desire to keep going wanes.

Track what matters to you. Track how you feel, how you're sleeping, your food, your steps, and your workouts. Take small steps and then add more. Give yourself time. Habits aren't created or changed overnight. Let's take our "Sugar Freedom" challenge as an example to demonstrate what Habit Shift can look like.

Sugar Freedom

Sugar. Too much sugar is literally a killer, but it's everywhere and in everything. Quitting sugar can feel almost impossible, and for good reason, it's a habit that touches most people's lives. From the dark chocolate before bed (no judgment) to the ice cream and Netflix, it's insidious. When I lead several Sugar Freedom events each year, the accountability texts fly when people are in the throes of sugar cravings! So instead of going cold turkey, this is where small habit shifts come in. I suggest starting with something simple like "no sugar after 7 pm." Eventually, this becomes a new habit, and there is an immediate win. You've given your brain a rule but not an unreasonable one. Then, you can shift again going forward.

When you do that, you take away the need to negotiate with yourself. When cravings start, you can simply say, sorry, it's after 7 pm, I can have a treat tomorrow if I want. The endless loop of negotiating (we always lose), the should I or shouldn't I, is removed. Awareness is key yet again. We always lose when we start negotiating with ourselves. Set a rule, remove the problem, and the issue resolves, just like the example that a phone next to you triggers the addiction (habit) to scroll mindlessly. Removing the trigger by creating a rule soothes the habit brain.

Speaking of soothing, learning to enlist the help of soothers; caffeine-free tea you elevate to a tea ritual, a bath, reading for enjoyment in a favorite spot, an evening walk, or better yet, a walk in the woods, a massage, whatever their special enjoyment makes habit shifting easier.

This is where curiosity comes in. In the sugar example, consider what could you possibly use to replace the sugar desire? Soothers come in a wide variety, but if you look closely at soothers, you'll notice all you've done is given your habit brain a small rule. This instead of that. And something different to enjoy. Seldom do people wake up the next morning thinking, "I can eat the sugary treat now." This is key - be aware of your habits and actions, then give yourself other options.

It's also good to remind yourself of the benefits of your habit shift. Such as, when you stop the evening sugar snacking, tell yourself you'll sleep better; better sleep leads to better movement, better movement leads to greater fitness and weight loss/muscle gain, and the cascading effect of good continues!

You need to understand your brain on habits and take control early before your brain does. Speaking of brains taking over, another issue that stops our fitness often before we even get started is our past! The excuses, the potential problems, the lack of motivation, and no one to lean on. These are real roadblocks, and in Part 3, we'll look at dismantling them for good. You'll finally have all the tools you need to get on track and stay there for good!

KEY TAKEAWAYS, ACTIONS, AND JOURNAL PROMPTS

Grab your Freedom Journal and take 5-10 minutes to brainstorm how you can apply habit shifting to your habits that currently stand in the way of your North Star and the life you desire. Follow this guide and see what ideas and solutions you can come up with!

Habit Shifting Quick Guide:

1. Desire. Is this something you truly desire?
2. Awareness. Become aware of your current habits.
3. Get curious. What's something different to try or do?
4. Plan. The simpler your plan, the better.
5. Act. Imperfect action is perfect.
6. Use all your senses. Immerse yourself in what you want.
7. Test & Track. And then test and track some more.
8. No self-judgment. Ever. This is a learning process, not a beatdown.
9. Time. It takes as long as it takes. Action today is better than no action at all!
10. Rinse and repeat

Wow, give yourself a high five and say congrats! You've done the hard work, and now it's time to focus on the shortcuts that will help you stay on track and get back on track with ease.

PART 3

CHAPTER 9
SMASHING EXCUSES

"The quickest way to change your life? Remove an excuse." -Kelly

Action Takers are my favorite women. The fact that you're already here, at chapter 9, tells me you are serious about your fitness future. Congratulations! In part three of this book, you'll find plenty of 'quick wins' to apply to your plan. Creating your fitness plan and then learning to habit shift is work. And you did it.

There's one small thing I'd like to address as we go forward…excuses. Excuses often look like reasonable issues. Let's go through some of the most common excuses I hear and how to smash those excuses one by one!

When I start working with a new client, something I need to know upfront is: "Why haven't they been focusing on their fitness?" The number one answer I get is, "I don't have the time." It can be hard to find the time. I get that. We're busy, everyone's busy. It feels like we can't fit one more thing in. But maybe fitting in more is not the answer.

The real answer is to do less of the things in life that don't matter and take our energy away.

No Time and Finding Time

Recall the previous chapter, and note that the way to start or shift a habit you WANT is awareness. *So become aware.* Look for your biggest time wasters. Spend a day watching what you do. If you want to get crazy serious, write down everything you do, minute by minute. Personally, I've never done this because I forget halfway through the day, but I can promise you, I take an audit every few months just to see what time wasters have crept in. I'm not talking about taking a book break or watching a movie. But if you feel like you don't have time, look at what you're doing that doesn't move you forward in life!

A couple of years ago, I was asked to contribute to a book called *Number One Habits for Entrepreneurs*. They asked me to give one habit that people should have and one habit people should abandon. The habit I suggested that people abandon is universal. It doesn't matter if you're an entrepreneur, if you work for someone else, or don't work at all. That habit almost everyone needs to ditch is *all the mindless time spent on our screens.*

Our phones are amazing technology, it's mind-boggling what they can do. And they are designed by some very smart people who want to win our attention. Add to that the fact that the more time we spend on our phones, the more of a habit they become. They bing, ding, and vibrate to get our attention and bring us back to them, over and over. It's an addiction.

I was shocked to find I use my phone more than I thought. When I went through my phone and checked my screen time numbers, oh my. A lot of that time is spent listening to podcasts and audiobooks while driving and working out, great. There was quite a bit of time using google maps to navigate around traffic, and then there was time spent fiddling around. Probably from when I grab a second cup of coffee in the morning, sit down, and pick up my phone. Clicking on email or Socials instead of journaling or whatever else I had planned for that particular time! Next thing I know ten, twenty, thirty minutes have slipped by, wasted and gone for good.

Is too much screen time a problem for you? Take the 'screen time test' and check your settings...what's your daily average number? Is it more than you thought it would be? Write that number in your freedom journal and then come back to it in a couple of months and see if you've made any improvements.

Here are a few suggestions for limiting phone time:

- Turn off your notifications
- Turn off your ringer
- Put it away - studies have shown that just having your phone in sight triggers you to look at it
- Limit your social scrolling by using something like "Feed Eradicator," which removes your feed and allows you to choose where you go on social instead of allowing the AI to serve you options
- Use Do Not Disturb hours. You can still set it to allow certain numbers through

Remember, when you pick up your phone, two things will happen. You'll be drawn into the desire to click around, and you'll need to use valuable willpower to put it back down!

We can acquire the same additions for TV. Watching TV to relax or turn your brain off works. But, it becomes a problem when you binge instead of doing something that moves the needle. Sidenote to this, some of my clients find ways to stretch or exercise while watching. This is one of those...if it works for you, do it, instances!

One of my clients would complain week after week that she didn't have time to stretch. When we started looking time, I asked her if she had watched TV.

She said, "Yes, but I like to watch TV, I'm not stopping."

I said, "You don't have to stop. But you would like to start stretching, wouldn't you? Why don't you make an agreement with yourself to stretch when you watch TV?" She laughed and said okay, like she thought we were kidding.

After a couple of weeks, she actually started stretching while watching and was excited as it started to work. She went so far as to decide that if she wasn't stretching, she couldn't watch TV. Her stretching started making her ultra-aware of her excessive TV habit. She spent a lot of time in front of the TV!

On our next call, she brought all of this up. I suggested she go back to her Freedom Journal, where we talked about habit shifting, and see what she had written in answer to the question:

If I mastered my fitness consistency, what would I be doing differently?

She wrote: *I would be finding time, instead of never having time, to enjoy more of the things I used to love doing like hiking, biking, and Dragon Boating. I would sit less and move more. I would do my stretching and mobility that I know I NEED to do, but never prioritize. If I did all these things, I'd have more energy and more fun instead of feeling like life was not as bright anymore, I'd be making my own sunshine!*

Wow - she knew exactly where she wanted to go, so we used this as the perfect start to focusing on some easy habit shifts. Instead of doing away completely with her TV shows, which was her first inclination, I suggested finding some small shifts that she could live with that weren't an all-or-nothing decision. We settled on finding three nights a week when she would seriously limit her TV (she still had time to watch a favorite show and stretch). She then made plans to use that time to do some of the things she missed doing. It wasn't a perfect solution because the timing wasn't always there, but the more she did it, the more she found ways to change her actions.

From no time to stretch to enough time to bring back things she loved doing. This is a perfect example of smashing excuses, taking actions that make the biggest results, and shifting habits to make life better. A win, win, win!

Here's a controversial waste for you, giving your time away. Benjamin Franklin said, "If you want something done, ask a busy person {woman}." We are so good at getting a lot done. As busy women, it's one of our superpowers. We take care of people, projects, and passions in our lives. And I think we need to learn to turn loose of some of these things so we can focus on ourselves. We need to become our own priority. That feels a little selfish, right? And we can't help anyone else if we don't feel good ourselves.

I challenge you to *look at any areas you are giving your time away and ask yourself; does this serve me, how is this improving my life, can I let this go?* When I was my mother's caretaker, I have to admit there were times I didn't want to do it, but I loved my mom dearly and knew it wouldn't last forever. There was another time when I was asked to head up a project that I had played a small part in previously. I felt it was my duty to step in and help. What I didn't know was I was stepping into a, quite frankly, viper pit. The people who were involved at the top level bickered and tried to push me around. They were not nice to play with! I did my part for two years and then turned in my resignation. My previous tormentors wailed and moaned. I stood firm, and as my life became simpler and I had more time, I was so grateful that I had let this responsibility go.

Another way to "find" time is to see what you can delegate or double time. Ever feel like you should do everything? Take care of the house. Buy the groceries. Care for those around us. Walk the dog. Yes, these are all important. And yes, some of these might be delegatable.

Where can you delegate in your life?

Grocery shopping. When the pandemic began, I started having my groceries delivered. I actually enjoy grocery shopping, but driving in a big city, especially when it seems all of Houston is also on the roads, makes it untenable. Driving to the store, shopping, and returning home could take me well over two hours. These days I frequently still opt for grocery delivery. That's two hours of my week back.

One of my clients takes time away from her company once a week to babysit and be with her grandson. She loved it and noticed that babysitting day was a "no exercise" day. She started wondering if she could double-time a walk and babysitting. It turns out that a quarter mile from where her grandson lived were some awesome trails. Now she gets to spend time with him and hiking. What a win!

Look for small ways to make time to start putting it towards your fitness.

'It's too hot. It's too cold.'

Another "I can't exercise" reason I hear from people is the weather. No judgment. I swear, every year, I'm shocked at how hot Houston summers are. I never learn! Weather can affect our fitness plans in two ways; short-term bad weather, too much rain, wind, etc., and seasonal weather issues; heat, snow, and ice.

Remember when planning your weekly workout for short-term weather issues: check the weather! If you're in a time of the year when the weather can be rocky, have options ready and be willing to move your schedule around. If you think your Pickleball or group hike might be canceled due to weather, this could look like having an indoor class like Pilates, yoga, or a video dance class.

For seasonal disturbances, be ready early!

Kim is a client in Houston. Because of heat sensitivity, she can't work out in the Houston summer heat. She'd do all of her outdoor exercisings through May. Then in June, she would switch to indoor classes for the next four months. After four months, she'd head back outside. Simple, except that when you get in a grove, it can be hard to change it up. For Kim, a cyclist, she could ride most of the fall, winter, and spring, and then all of a sudden, the heat would happen. Surprised (see, I'm not the only one. :) She would stop cycling and suddenly forget how to switch it up. When she came to me during the pandemic, her indoor classes were closed, and she felt lost.

This was a simple two-step process. First, I had her purchase an indoor trainer that hooked directly to her bike. She's never tried one before but found she really enjoyed it. Second, since she spent so much time cycling, I suggested that she find a second or even third form of cardio and that she absolutely needed to add some resistance. Now she has added pilates year-round, summer is her building period for resistance training, and the remainder of the year is her maintenance phase.

Dee, who lived up north, came to me because it was too cold to exercise outside in the winter. Her exercise of choice was running, but icy conditions were dangerous. Her fitness was slipping, and she was panicking.

I asked her, is it too cold for you to have fun outside?

After a pause, she replied, *"I don't mind the cold, I just don't want to fall running."*

So we switched it up. Now she does a lot of snowshoeing and cross-country skiing. She said, *"You know, I always kind of thought that snowshoeing and even cross-country skiing was going to be lame, and that's why I never tried it. I'm working so many more muscles than I ever did running, and I've actually got a butt now, in a good way now!"* Plus, she's having fun.

Ask yourself, what can I do that would be so much fun that I would make it a priority and find the time and desire? That's one of the many ways you become consistent with your fitness. When fitness becomes fun, you have time for it, it's a priority, and you'll drop the excuses and get moving.

'I'm Too Tired'

Do you ever catch yourself using the "I'm too tired" excuse? If you're constantly feeling tired, then you need to know why. Do you need to get tested by your doctor for potential problems? Do you need better sleep? To eat more or differently?

Often times I see the "I'm too tired" excuse vanish when people start exercising. Exercise doesn't make you tired (with possibly the exception of long bouts of cardio or training sessions). Exercise typically makes you more energized! Even if you're starting with slow walks, those slow walks will get you going.

'I'm Just Not Motivated'

One last excuse to address is the "I'm just not motivated" excuse. Honestly? This is like nails on a blackboard to me - LOL. Motivation comes from everything we've been discussing so far in this book. It comes from having a North Star and returning to it when you're not motivated. It comes from moving; a body in motion stays in motion. It comes from tracking so that you can see results. Motivation is made, not something you either have or you don't. Yes, some people are naturally more driven, but even with those people I stop and wonder, is it something they are born with or something they've created in their lives? Make motivation a part of who you are!

Fit is Freedom Friends - Lynn

She had worked very hard her entire life, her business was financially successful, and her kids were out of the house. She had this dream to play more, do more, travel, and have adventures around the world. But, man, was she busy. She was the head of a local Foundation and a leader in her church and in her community. She was the person everyone turned to when they needed anything because she knew how to get things done.

But there was one little problem, she was running out of motivation. At an impasse, she realized that she wanted more time and fun for herself. Having always thought that she was just a "Naturally motivated person," she was starting to understand her motivation had come from enjoying what she was doing. Overwhelmed, she realized that everyone wanted something from her, and she didn't see a way to have the playtime she wanted for herself.

She was burned out and unmotivated.

We came up with a list of everything that was overwhelming her, and at the very core of that list were all her extra obligations. Her business could run with very little input from her. Her kids were doing fine, and financially she was set.

So the big question became...In a perfect world, how would her life change?

It just so happened that since she'd been the leader in all her outside-of-work endeavors for such a very long time, she felt ok stepping away from the reins. There was a little guilt there, but it was also time to let other people take their turn.

She picked an end date for all her volunteer endeavors. She made checklists and systems; knowing her, she probably even made videos on how to do everything! And then, she took action and started letting people know that she was no longer available to manage all these projects.

A very big, courageous step!

I wasn't privy to her conversations, but I'm willing to bet everyone secretly couldn't believe she had helped them for as long as she had!

In our previous discussion, she was just about wrapping up the remaining aspects of a fundraising initiative, eagerly mapping out her future endeavors of play, travel, extended hiking excursions, and rigorous training for thrilling adventure trips. It's incredible how she transitioned from being confined and immobilized, with limited opportunities to pursue her passions, to now leading a life infused with thrilling escapades. All of this was made possible because she dared to ask herself the pivotal questions and wholeheartedly embraced the power of listening and adaptation.

In the next chapter, we'll be looking at accountability and how to use it correctly. Used right, it's a powerful tool. Used wrong, it's nothing but a disappointing time waster! Before we dive into all things accountability, you'll want to do this one quick exercise so you can 10X your accountability partner results. Grab your Freedom Journal, and let's do an 'excuse deep dive' together, given in the prompt box.

KEY TAKEAWAYS, ACTIONS, AND JOURNAL PROMPTS

Excuse Deep-Dive:

When we don't have what we want in life, one of the pieces that hold everyone back are our excuses for why we can't have what we say we want.

Let's find an excuse that's holding you back from your fitness and adventure dreams, and bust it! Time for a little journaling (and if you're thinking you don't have time for this, this might be a good excuse to start with:)

Q1. Pick one thing you say you want to have or do.

_____

_____

_____

Q2. What's stopping you?

Free-write for a couple of minutes, what's everything that's holding you back from having exactly what you want. Is it no time, your relationship, where you live, lack of clarity, or lack of finances, what's stopping you? List it all out.

Q3. In a perfect world, how would this change?

Get crazy. Come up with silly ideas, new ideas, all ideas. Reach for the stars. What could you do differently?

Q4. Pick one idea and run with it. Give it a chance before you discount it!

_____

_____

_____

CHAPTER 10
ACCOUNTABILITY: THE GOOD, THE BAD, AND THE STOP IT RIGHT NOW!

"Accountability makes your fitness path easier - but ONLY if it's the right kind of accountability. If you go with the popular choices, you'll set yourself up to fail."- Kelly

Ask most people what the golden arrow is regarding fitness consistency, and they'll say, "Accountability. Having accountability buddies. That's what will keep me on track."

There are many studies that show that an accountability buddy can increase follow-through by more than 70%. People fail to understand that it's not just having an accountability buddy but having the right KIND of accountability buddy that matters. And that's what this chapter is all about.

A body in motion stays in motion, and having a buddy will keep you moving. The pitfalls happen when you pick the wrong type of buddy!

Let me ask you - who would be your go-to accountability buddy; your best friend, your life partner, or your dog? Pick your dog because, one way or another, the dog walk will happen! But if you don't have a dog, don't worry, dogs aren't even on my list of best accountability buddies. Before we look at becoming 100% accountable to ourselves, let's look at the BIG BAD 3 of accountability: your life partner, your best friend, and the latest and greatest app. All accountability is not created equal!

Big Bad One: Your Partner

Your partner knows your triggers, your hot buttons, and what to say when to get the result they want. If your partner isn't 100% down on your fitness plan, food choices, or getting up early to train for that fitness vacation, you're in trouble. They know when you're at your weakest and how to gently suggest how much more fun it would be to skip the walk and grab a pizza and the remote. Or bring home that bottle of wine at the end of a long hard day when they know damn well you said you wanted to skip the wine for a month (or the chocolate cake - insert your kryptonite). Your partner knows how to get out of any fitness plan you rope them into.

Fit is Freedom Friend Suzie - And the Reluctant Accountability Partner

Suzie was a friend of a friend. We started talking at a dinner party, and she told me everything that was going on. A recent injury led to surgery which led to muscle loss and weight gain, which led to depression. She was pretty down in the dumps when our mutual friend introduced us. We chatted, and as she told me her story, I couldn't help but give her a couple of ideas. She became really excited and exclaimed, *"This is awesome, I'm going to get Doug to join me, and we'll get back on track together!"* I didn't say anything, but by the looks Doug was sending our way, I wasn't sure he was all in on this.

About a month went by, and as I was checking my 1:1 appointments for the next day, I saw Suzie on my calendar. Awesome! I was excited to chat and see how they were doing. Well, actually, they weren't doing anything at all. As we went over what wasn't working, I heard a consistent sentence, *"You know, we work so hard, and when Doug suggests going out for dinner and drinks instead of me having to make dinner at home, I just say yes. But then we always go for the comfort food."*

Together, we came up with a new plan for her (and Doug), which included a lot of meal planning early in the week and morning exercise instead of the afternoon exercise they kept meaning to do. She scheduled another call in one month, and off she went with her new plan. She was excited, but my guess was that he couldn't be, but I crossed my fingers, hoping I'd be wrong.

On our next call, I could tell she was back where she started and super frustrated. This was the conversation I was hoping we wouldn't be having. I suggested she let Doug do whatever he wanted to do for his own health and fitness and solely focus on herself. *"But what if he never gets back in shape, what will I do?"* I guess you'll just have to let him be his own adult because right now, it's not working for either of you, and it's dragging you down.

We re-made her plan and got her into the Fit is Freedom accountability community. It was hard for her because she naturally was a very giving and loving woman who wanted the best for both of them. But she couldn't make him do anything he wasn't ready for.

Can you guess what happened? With the right kind of accountability, it was easy for Suzie to start focusing on her own health. She started feeling and looking great. And, of course, the more she focused on getting her fitness back, the more interested Doug became in doing the same.

These days they take active trips together but don't depend on each other to get them moving and training!

Keep them as your partner and enlist a more appropriate accountability buddy!

Big Bad Two: Your Best Friends

Have you ever enlisted your best friend in a fitness goal? That friend you totally connect with, who's busy and successful just like you? At first, you're both super excited to get started on your new fitness goals. The texts and emojis are flying, conversations are flowing, and someone misses a day. And then another day. And then one more. What do you do? Conversation fades, and it gets quieter until you both just tiptoe away. She might be the best friend in the world, but because she is, she's the worst kind of accountability buddy. A best friend's job is to make you feel good, to support you through thick and thin, not to tell you to get off your backend and get to the gym or put down the ice cream. She feels your pain and wants you to feel better, **whatever it takes**.

Good friends let each other off the hook. They support each other with love, but not tough love. More like, "You didn't work out this morning? It's ok, you have a lot on your plate right now…maybe we should catch up over drinks, and we can start again next week…."

A Personal Story

I have a very dear friend who was fairly athletic. She was a swimmer and ran 10K and half-marathons. And then she bought a floundering company and became hell-bent on turning it around, fast! She did a great job, and within about two and a half years, the company had become profitable. But at what cost? Over those two point five years, she completely quit exercising, her meals had become take-out, taken in front of her computer most days and evenings. She developed aches and pains she'd never had before, gained about thirty pounds, and her sleep was crap. We'd occasionally talk, and I'd ask her if she was running or doing anything. She always replied, *"I'll start next month when we're a little more profitable."*

And then I got the call.

"I'm in trouble! I feel like hell, nothing, absolutely nothing, fits me anymore, and the doctor said I was pre-diabetic. Will you help me get back on track?"

I bet you know how the story went. :) We started off great that first week. Text check-ins were checked off, and workouts were solid. Week two started out a little rocky, she had a bunch of appointments on Monday and Tuesday but was back on track Wednesday. But then, week three rolled around.

I texted her to see what her schedule was for the week. Crickets.

So that afternoon, I sent text number two, "How's it going?"

I waited two days and sent a third text filled with lots of emojis and exclamation points, "How you doing, How can I help, what's going on…."

The next day I called. To her credit, she did pick up the phone, and we chatted. The bottom line was she didn't feel like she had time at that moment to get back in shape. I might help people be fitness accountable and consistent for my living, but I'm no different than any other good friend. Of course, she got a 100% free pass, and when she asked if we could have dinner instead of texting about exercise, I agreed. We ate copious amounts of Italian food, drank good wine, and laughed for hours. I was reminded that best friends are friends first and NOT accountability buddies.

A month later, I got a text "Can we start doing check-ins again?"

I invited her to dinner and gave her the number of an excellent fitness coach I know. Best friends should be just that. We've all had it happen, your friend starts fit-fading, and she doesn't show up or text you her workouts. The updates end, and so does your accountability.

Big Bad Three: Apps or Tracking Devices

Tracking devices and apps can be great for recording what you do but not for holding you accountable. They may work for a little while, but a lot less than we are led to believe. In fact, one health and wellness company said they found that after someone downloaded their fitness app, it was used on average 3-5 times TOTAL, and then app usage would stop almost completely. When customers were asked later on a follow-up survey if they had used the app, the most common response was, "I can imagine using it." Imagining doesn't get you where you want to be. It's not your fault. Digital buddies are easily out-of-sight-out-of-mind.

Interestingly, apps can also backfire on us. Since they are designed to give our brain a dopamine hit whenever we get a 'like' or a 'cheer' from the group chat or app itself, when we stop following or checking in, that shot of dopamine disappears. This makes people feel even more down and disheartened than before they started.

So how do you make accountability work for and not against you? Use what I term; Layered Accountability.

Layered Accountability

Layered accountability doesn't depend on only one particular action. You make a more substantial foundation when you use several options or a layered approach. The fact that it's "layered" means you have accountability in multiple ways, making it harder to escape or avoid! Especially when you utilize what truly appeals and isn't a cookie-cutter suggestion. Keep mixing and matching your accountability until you find your personal style. Here's an example of what one of my clients uses:

Karen's Layers of Accountability:

- Written schedule on her office wall AND in her online calendar
- Clothes and gear out the night before and where she sees it when she gets up
- She has friends who she invites to 5K's with but not to her training days. She's found as much as she loves her friends, they're unreliable and frequently look for ways out of training. If they don't make it to the 5K, she goes anyway
- She located a group of women hikers who post hikes weekly, she joins their hikes
- She tracks her movement with a Fitbit and MapMyRun
- She keeps a monthly calendar that she marks off her movement and training so she can see her progress

Fit is Freedom Friend Joy - Layered Accountability in Action

Before we started working together, my client, Joy, a ridiculously busy business owner, was burning the candle at both ends. She had health issues that were slowing her down, and weight gain and less flexibility were getting her down emotionally, physically, and mentally! She was utilizing the app, Strava, in an attempt to stay on track during the week as she typically worked long days and felt drawn in numerous ways. She didn't really like the app (nothing against the Stravia, some people love it). It had never become a habit she embraced. She thought it would give her the accountability she was looking for, but it felt like a big void that she would post to, but no one responded. She had friends on the app, but no one was paying attention to help her with the accountability she so dearly desired. Ultimately the app and her workouts fell to the wayside.

Because she had already been using the app and was used to it, I encouraged her to revisit the app and add me to her list when we started working together. Now she knew someone was watching her actions and results.

Next, she joined the Fit is Freedom community, which gave her real-time text accountability with a group of fitness-focused women. Community was something she had wished for, for a very long time. It was an exciting addition, knowing she had friends and cheerleaders who had her back! She also enrolled in monthly 1:1 coaching calls with me and weekly check-ins on the group coaching calls. All these steps may sound like a considerable amount of time, but, except for the coaching, it took approximately five-ten minutes maximum out of her day.

Finally, to cement her commitment, she joined us on a Hiking Retreat, which meant training was required! She nailed it.

As she moved forward with her layered accountability plan, Joy had a revelation in just a short few months. As enjoyable as all the accountability was, it became something that was fun and not necessary. She had become accountable to herself.

The Power of Personal Accountability

Another way to look at layered accountability is to think of it as a fitness pyramid, with the simplest, most basic options at the base of the pyramid and moving up with more definitive and hands-on options.

Step one is the base of the pyramid and is something simple. It could be an online challenge, or a fitness app like Strava or My Fitness Pal, one that incorporates gamification, is a plus. Step two is to add a fitness community of like-minded women. Consider an online or a local group of people who enjoy similar activities, a meet-up, or even a neighborhood group. Search for activities you enjoy or would like to learn to do, like hiking, pickleball, or cycling groups. Step three is to find a structured option like a coach, a personal trainer, or specific classes. Step four is to plan a personal challenge. It could be an adventure travel trip, a specific hike, a bike ride, or learning a new activity, how can you challenge yourself and get excited at the same time?

Finally, at the very top of that pyramid is you! In the end, you're the person who's going to be the most responsible for what happens in your life. One of the most overlooked pieces of advice when it comes to accountability is to master the role that you play. When you become your own best accountability partner, your fitness becomes a breeze.

When you learn to be accountable to yourself, you step into your true personal power.

Here are a few suggestions to make yourself more personally accountable. Grab your Freedom Journal and decide which one of these you're going to use. (Hint: pick a few, multiple options make it easier to stay accountable to yourself)

Shortcuts to Personal Accountability

- Personal awareness. What really engages you? Is it results, routine, tracking, seeing changes, and improvement? Probably all of the above! How do you measure that?

- Track and measure exactly what action you take and your progress

- Schedule it. What is scheduled is real.

- Visuals: Post your schedule where you will see it (which you should have by now), track your progress where you can be reminded, and put a calendar on your wall. When you see your schedule and your progress, it will encourage you to keep going.

- Plan something to work toward and give yourself a time-specific goal or, my favorite - pick something to train for.
- Try something new. What's something you've always wanted to do? Do it.
- Awareness. Pay attention to what motivates and drives you, and then use it.
- Don't focus on the 'shoulds'; this pulls our energy down. Focus on what you want and what you have achieved so far.
- Celebrate (for longer than just 20 seconds) before you move on to what's next.
- Visualize and journal to keep your dreams and desires alive.

Accountability helps you create habits and cements those habits so that you can take action and trust yourself without needing outside help as much. There is nothing wrong with external accountability, but the more you depend on yourself, the easier it becomes to do what you need to do and keep taking the actions you need repeatedly. Ready to layer your accountability? Grab your freedom journal, go back through the chapter, and pick 2-3 accountability steps you can use today. Write them down and find ways to apply them in your life, ASAP!

Layered accountability can move the needle when it comes to fitness consistency. But, sometimes, we need a little push or a quick win. In the next chapter, I'll share my toolbox filled with quick wins and easy tools to keep you motivated and moving toward your North Star!

CHAPTER 11
THE TOOLBOX

> *"Every single one of us can use a little help at one time or another. Having the right tools to choose from makes help a breeze."* - Kelly

Motivation can seem like something you're either born with or you just don't have it. The truth? It's not one thing. It's a compilation of many things; learned behavior, energy levels, desire, and so much more. And I'm here to tell you in this chapter that you can shortcut the need for motivation when you have the right tools! There are times when every single person has less than zero motivation. When that happens, it's time to use one or several quick-start strategies to get you back on track and moving again. I designed these tools to be quick, easy to grab, and even easier to apply. We don't have time to waste if we feel a "wallow" coming on!

But first, before you start grabbing tools out of the box, make sure you have these three foundational steps in place;

1. Your 'why' (remember the North Star), 2. the beginning of a fitness plan, and 3. personal awareness so you're ready when excuses show up. Once you have the framework in place, use these strategies to keep you moving in the right direction!

13 Tools to Kickstart and Fuel Your Motivation!

#1 Schedule

At the risk of sounding like a broken record, you need a schedule. What is scheduled is real. If it's a passing idea in your mind, that's all it is. Everyone has a different method of scheduling. You have to use what is right for you. Some examples of scheduling tools:

- Wall calendar
- Online calendar
- Work Calendar
- Post it notes
- Freedom Journal
- Fitness App/Tracker

You have to use what works for you!

I'd like to tell a story about myself. For years, and I mean years, I've used this (now ratty) dry-erase board that has one week on it. Nothing else, just Week of: and then squares. I have used this through training for numerous events and challenges over the years, and it always served me. I'd add my weekly workouts, rest days, mobility, scheduled fun activities, and wildcard days. Every day I'd check off what I got done, take note of what I missed, and move things around if needed. Earlier this year, I decided I was tired of looking at that board. Of course, I didn't really NEED it. I'd been at this fitness thing long enough that I could keep my schedule with a quick notation in my online calendar - easy peasy. I took it down, hung a beautiful photo in its place, and felt smug.

About two months later, I noticed that I wasn't hitting my usual 85-90% of what I had scheduled. In fact, I was hitting only 70% on some weeks. Not good! What was wrong with me?

I did a quick awareness scan and realized the problem - my dry-erase week, my security blanket was no longer there! I panicked a bit as I dug through my supply closet, wondering if I'd tossed it! But no, there it was, gathering dust in the corner. Down came the photo, up went my board, and I was back on track.

Find what works for you and stick to it (Kelly:)

#2 Something to look forward to/to train for

I typically have something on the horizon to train for. Be it an adventure retreat I'm leading, a race, or anything that challenges me, I like to know that there's a specific reason for training. We need something tangible to look forward to!

I was reminded of how powerful this tool is on the first hiking retreat I led for my inner circle. Everyone pulled together. They were excited and a little worried. Having the challenge and the fun of the upcoming retreat gave everyone a little extra push to stay on track. They had a goal that was past their comfort zone but oh so desirable. For many, the trip was a big scary hiking goal that motivated them and moved them in the right direction. What may have seemed insurmountable at the onset became manageable as everyone got in the groove of training virtually. It was hard work but so rewarding. The retreat gave everyone something to look forward to. This was such a successful training strategy that I now hold several adventure retreats each year. With an online training program, virtual accountability buddies, and a shared goal, everyone who participates - wins! The fact that we can come together in person after training makes these retreats even sweeter! When you're done reading and if you're interested in joining us on a retreat, stop by www.FitisFreedom.com/retreat and put your name on the list!

But not everyone wants to go on an adventure retreat - I get it! Here are some other ways you can use this tool. Plan an active family vacation or outing. One of the women in my inner circle has a godson who recently reached an age where he can participate in more energetic activities with her. She has made a plan to take her godson on an active camping trip that includes biking and hiking. She's doing everything necessary to be ready for that trip! A friend of mine is teaching her nieces and nephews how to skate. She looks forward to the days she takes them to the roller rink, and between rink sessions, she's working on her mobility and flexibility so she can lead the pack.

Maybe you've joined the pickleball craze or signed up for a "K" 5/10/25. Great, time to get in shape so it's enjoyable. One quick word of wisdom, give yourself time. If you haven't been active or actively training, assume you'll need a minimum of three months to get closer to where you want to be!

#3 Track

Let's gect tracking out of the way right away! This is one of the least liked or acted-on tools in the toolbox and is probably one of the top three most valuable tools.

What you track is personal, and it has to be something that: 1. Matters to you 2. Is not complicated to track. You'll find a couple of editable trackers in your book bonus section. Use these or use whatever works for you, but track what counts!

You might track your workouts, weights, how long you can stand on one leg, what you eat, or your protein intake. What makes tracking so powerful is looking back and seeing where you came from.

I asked one of my clients once to track her pushups. These weren't military, nose-to-the-floor pushups but slant pushups – something you do off a desk. She couldn't do a single slant push-up when we first started. After about a month, she could do 37 pushups. That's huge! The funny part was she wasn't tracking her pushups at first, but I was. When she saw the massive increase in strength and ability, it lit a fire, and she started tracking for herself. Her wins kept her ignited.

Tracking gives you visible results, especially if the numbers on the scale* aren't going down.

Suggestions on what to track:

- Inches instead of weight
- Perceived effort and how you improve in a class, a trail, a ride
- Bone mass increase with a DEXA scan
- Weights used and reps done
- Food count; protein, carbs, and calories

*A note about using the scale to track: My only caveat is to skip the daily scale weigh-in. Our body changes daily. If you must use the scale, do it one day a week. Promise yourself and me that if the number fluctuates a couple of pounds, you won't panic. I can't tell you how many times someone has told me they gained 2-3 pounds over a weekend. It's not physically possible to gain 2-3 pounds of fat or muscle over a weekend. It is possible to have a couple of pounds of water weight that comes from what you eat, dehydration (!), hormones, and where you are in your monthly cycle. Scales tend to bring us down because our weight fluctuates. It fluctuates. What we eat, water weight, bloating, and even dehydration affect our weight, but it doesn't matter.

#4 FPA: Friggin Plan Ahead

I mentioned FPA earlier in the book, let's deep dive and learn to embrace it because FPA can be one of the most essential tools you have! It's a motto in the Fit is Freedom Community… Just FPA. Let's just say that stands for friggin' plan ahead. Planning ahead is your superpower. And everyone (including me) at some point thinks they don't need it.

Here's how FPA works:

1. Schedule your movement
2. The evening before, put out everything you'll need for what's on your schedule. If you're going to the gym, have your workout clothes out, your shower supplies, your gym bag - whatever you need.
3. Pro Tip: don't put your supplies into your bag - place them in front of your bag where you can see everything and see what's missing. I learned this skill years ago when I was doing small triathlons. At each race, you had limited space for all your gear, and you needed that gear to be easily accessible. The night before the race, I would put out all my gear and then check and recheck. Placing everything I needed on a small towel was the ultimate FPA. I was prepared and never surprised. When I quit racing, I got lazy and would find myself forgetting things, thus taking way too long to get out the door in the morning for my exercise. When I brought back the FPA, I'd be out the door in a flash, never worrying, "Did I forget {insert everything you worry about forgetting}!"

I have a client who leaves for work very early in the morning, and she was forgetting her workout clothes, even though they were right by the door on her way out. So, in FPA fashion, she filled her gym bag and put it in her car the night before. She quit missing her workouts!

For me, when I plan on going for a long hike or bike ride, I fill up and put out my water bottles, snacks, hat, sunscreen, sunglasses, and whatever I might need, the night before. If I know I'll be hiking, biking, or moving for longer than a few hours, I make a protein shake the night before and put it in a small cooler. That way, when I am stumbling around in the morning, I don't have to think. I just grab it and go. By planning ahead, I save myself a lot of time and typically don't forget anything, especially if I "stage everything."

So FPA my friend, you'll save time, worry and have more fun!

#5 Invest in Yourself

When we commit financially, we have a bigger stake in the game. Whether it's a trainer, a coach, or classes, sign up. For years I had a personal trainer. Between the appointment on my calendar and the monthly prepayment, I was guaranteed to make it to the session. Well spent money.

How much you spend is completely open. You don't want it to be so much that you're always ready to quit if you miss a class or so little that it doesn't matter. My friend joined a gym that was only $12 a month. In her mind, even if she didn't go, it didn't matter. She would never miss the $12.

When I asked her how the gym was going, she said, "You know what? I never go to that gym, I don't really care about the $12, but I keep paying, and maybe I'll go someday." The financial output wasn't enough to get her attention.

On the flip side, I had been wanting to try a new Pilates studio. It was a lot more each month than I was used to spending, and I did everything possible to get to that class. But, after three months and a lot of money, I realized it wasn't worth it. I was stressing about getting my money's worth and jumping through hoops to get to the classes. It wasn't worth the worry.

#6 Visual Reminders

Visual reminders are another great way to stay motivated. One visual reminder could be the schedule board you keep on the wall, where you can see it every day. Post-it notes are another example. I use Post-its all the time. I'll write something like, "Congratulations on finishing your 25k." I love Post-its because you can move them around to different spots. If you leave them in the same place, you will stop seeing them.

I also like using vision boards. You can put all your plans, dreams, and desires you want for yourself on vision boards. This year, I did something a little different and created an adventure vision board. On my adventure board, I put a multi-sport trip to Costa Rica, kayaking the Smoky Mountains, hiking in Montana, surfing in San Diego, and eating in Italy :). I may not make every trip on my board, but just looking at it gets me excited and motivated to workout more!

I had so much fun putting it together, the excitement keeps bringing me back to my WHY. It also just gave me something to do when I had time off from an injury and couldn't do anything else for two weeks. I stayed focused and ready for when I could get back in the game.

If you love a to-do list, checking your items off your list can be a great booster. I have my schedule next to my desk on a dry-erase board, and I check off what I do each day. Doing this gives me that little boost of endorphins and dopamine that makes me think, "I did this, and tomorrow's going be even better."

One of my clients prints off a monthly calendar. Her goal is to do some movement every day, and as she crosses off each day that she succeeds, her determination grows! At the time of writing this, we've worked together for five months, and she has five calendars to show. At the top of each calendar, she writes her weight, her waist measurement, how many box step-ups she can do, and how long she can stand on one leg with her eyes closed. Each month the numbers get better, and her excitement grows. Today, at 63, she is in better shape than ever; she's strong, flexible, and excited about what's next!

#7 External Positive Input

Listen to and read things that get you going. It could be music, a podcast, audiobooks, a motivational book, or maybe a great health book. This is one of my favorite things to do when I'm training. If I need a little extra push, I put in my earbuds, turn on my coach or a podcast, and get moving.

There are podcasts about fitness, mindset, well-being, happiness, whatever it is that will get you motivated. If you're part of the Fit is Freedom experience, you have a hundred fitness audios and videos inside the course. Consider listening to an audiobook if you want to turn off your brain and not think about your exercise.

It really doesn't matter what you use. Just find something that gives you the extra push you need that day.

#8 Accountability Buddies

We covered accountability buddies in depth in the previous chapter, but just to reiterate, accountability buddies work as long as they're the right kind! Having an accountability option in your toolbox is very powerful, especially when you hit a wall or are in a slump. Real accountability buddies create a true level of accountability, they must be people and groups who have your back and can gently call you out when needed.

The final outcome you are reaching for is to be 100% accountable to yourself and to have that buddy on speed dial when you catch yourself floundering!

#9 Motivation Multipliers: Celebrate, Declutter & the Alphabet Game

The term Motivation Multipliers comes from my *Consistency is Key* program. There are twelve multipliers inside the program. I'll cover three of my faves here.

Number one is to **celebrate.** Celebrate the small wins as much as the big ones. It's one of the top things I work with my clients on. We typically don't celebrate our wins. We're so driven to hit that next goal that we give the goal we just achieved a passing nod and then drive ourselves forward for what's next.

Stop chasing and start celebrating the wins that you have.

A week after I finished my 25k, I realized I had never even thought about celebrating. I just checked that one off and went on to my next goal. What the heck!?! That was a hard race, and even though I felt like I was dead last in that race (I wasn't :) I finished and actually did pretty well. I never stopped to say to myself, "Wow. Congratulations, Kelly. You just did a really big thing!"

When I realized I had completed a big goal on my list, I stopped and acknowledged what I had done. I hadn't trained like I wanted to or checked the course before going (I probably would have bailed), but I did step up and do the race. After acknowledging my win, I made an appointment for a massage and lunch out with a friend. It was fun celebrating. We don't do it enough! Celebrate reaching your goals, however big or small you might think they are. You did it.

On a group call for my Sugar Freedom program, I asked the women to share their wins from the last weekend. Silence. As I looked around, a couple of them said, "Well, you know I didn't hit any big goals."

I drilled down. Surely everyone must have had at least one win?

Someone in the group said, "Well, I didn't have any wine, that's been bothering me this entire program. I feel good." Huge!

Someone else said, "I stopped drinking Coke." Another big win.

Sometimes we need to stop and check in to find those wins and pay attention. Celebrate and enjoy!

Another motivation multiplier is **decluttering**. Decluttering isn't very sexy like some motivators, but try it! When things are neat, clean, clear, and uncluttered, we have less to occupy our minds, and we can put our attention elsewhere. I believe decluttering is a superpower.

I have a personal example of decluttering to share. I think I'm a pretty neat person and keep things in good order…but one morning, I went to get a sports bra from the drawer and couldn't find even one. The drawer for my workout clothes and gear looked like clothes had exploded. So I stopped, gave myself 15 minutes, and got everything folded and back into place. Now when I need a sports bra or a workout shirt, I know exactly what drawer it will be in, laid out perfectly. No stress, no fuss, just easy and quick.

When you declutter your environment, it helps remove the clutter in your mind. Clarity can be another superpower, and decluttering can be a path to it! Decluttering allows you ease, making life more grab-and-go. Try it. It doesn't matter what you declutter, but once you start, it gets easier and the more you do it, the more space you will find in your life. The secret to decluttering is to go small. Pick a drawer instead of the entire wardrobe. One drawer will lead to another. It can almost be a moving meditation; a cup of coffee or tea, a little quiet music, and one more drawer is under your control.

The last motivation multiplier I want to share is **the alphabet game**. This motivator came about one day when I was doing a long bike ride. I was alone and probably an hour and a half into the ride and suddenly felt totally bored. I wanted to stop right there. If you're not a cyclist, you may not know this, but riding with earbuds is frowned upon from a safety standpoint (this could actually be said for most exercise outside, but this is for another time). So I'm riding along, nothing in my ears, and boredom sets in. But I was following a training plan and needed that long ride as much as I needed a distraction! It was time to get back on track.

The Alphabet Game:

Step 1 - Start by picking a theme. Let's use the example of Motivation.

Step 2 - Begin with the letter "A" and come up with a word that starts with the letter A that fits your theme. How about Action? Next, the letter "B" how about Big Goals (so what if it's two words, you're making up the rules here:) C could be Commitment, and so on. I've found that the combination of getting your mind interested, a good theme, and the willingness to keep moving forward makes the alphabet game a winner when you need a diversion!

#10 Rewards

Do you reward yourself? We often think that completing the action is reward enough. It becomes a "should." That's nice, but sometimes when there's a carrot dangling in front of us as a reward, it makes us a little more motivated. Rewards can be anything. A reward I frequently use is getting to go kayaking after finishing all the work I had on my list for that week. It's easy to think, "Well, I got all that done, maybe I should do a little more," but I've found when I honor grab-and-go myself, I come home energized and ready to tackle more instead of being tired from a long week.

Think about something that works for you as a reward. It could be buying yourself a new outfit, a massage, time off, a special dinner, or extra time to relax. Let's say you've just finished an entire training series you've been working on. Reward yourself and go buy that new pair of shoes you've been wanting. What are your rewards going to be? Think of a few and write them down. I write my rewards on Post-its and put them where I'm bound to see them. It keeps me on track and motivated.

#11 The 10-20-30

When you don't feel like exercising, or you're super busy and just don't see how you can fit anything else in your day, try a 10-20-30. The idea behind the 10-20-30 is that a body in motion stays in motion. So tell yourself you'll do whatever you had on your fitness schedule, but only for ten minutes. That's all you commit to. At the end of the 10 minutes, if you want to quit, then quit. You did what you said you were going to do.

Or, if at the end of your 10 minutes, you feel like you can go a little longer, do 20 minutes. Again, if after 20 minutes you still have some juice and feel like doing a little more, do 30 minutes.

The key is to give yourself permission to quit at 10, 20, or 30 minutes, with no judgment. You have permission to keep going if you want. Often, you'll find that the simple action of moving will motivate you to keep going.

#12 Tool: Make it fun

If it's not fun (at least some of the time), it's not sustainable. Fun comes in many forms. Consider these two sides of fun.

1. What you do

2. How you feel/think about what you're doing

What you're doing

Fun is subjective; what might be "fun" for a long-distance runner may be completely different than what you think of as fun. Maybe you love to dance and find that fun. For me, with three left feet, dancing is more stressful than fun. Find your own fun. Sprinkle them in your weekly schedule, add them to your calendar, PLAN for fun, don't hope it will just happen! Have something to look forward to. Quick, grab your freedom journal and make a list of 5-10 things that you would like to do, like to learn to do, like to try, and start sprinkling them into your life.

I was on a call with one of my awesome clients. She has literally knocked all her goals out of the park over the last year, and she was searching for what was next but really just wanted a little break. We devised a few small fun things to try over the summer. She would stick to her usual workout schedule and sprinkle these in over a couple of months:

1. Spin class

2. Rock wall climbing

3. A reformer Pilates class

4. Yoga class (bonus points for outdoor yoga)

5. Barre Class

6. Bowling

7. Pickleball

8. And Zipline if she was feeling wild!

What a fun list of things to try over the summer!

How about you? What's your list of fun activities going to be? If you're not having fun, you will lose interest. Excitement kills boredom every time. Whether it's a new kind of exercise, a new activity, or signing up for a class, find something that is fun for you or you always wanted to try. Fitness freedom is about so much more than just going to the gym. It's truly about all the fun you can have with your fit and healthy body!

How you feel/think about what you're doing:

My client had wanted to find something extra fun to do over the upcoming weekend to help herself through a tough time, but the weather wasn't cooperating. She'd texted me a few of her ideas, but she was basically in a major storm situation. And then I got a video text from her. She was soaking wet in a parking garage and cracking up. Basically, her video said, "I found my joy today but didn't think it would be climbing the stairs in a parking garage soaking wet. But I did it, and I'm having a blast."

That's how to choose mind over matter and get moving, find something you can do, and then enjoy it in the moment!

#13 Beginner's Mind

When we're used to being super accomplished, successful women. It can be hard to start small and embrace a beginner's mind. :) We expect to be good at what we try and to be able to keep up with everyone else. It doesn't always work that way. So many things I've learned (or am still learning) over the years I need a beginner's mind; when I started cycling, distance skating, sailing, whitewater kayaking, surfing, SUP…you name it, anything I have tried that was effort also required beginner's mind. The willingness to not be the best, to not know what you're doing, to really suck at first! If it matters to you or is fun, drop your ego. Adopt a curious, beginner mind and just have fun!

Fit is Freedom Friend - Shonda

Shonda had never done much exercise her entire life. She was in her early sixties and had been doctor-scared into getting into shape. She was overwhelmed about where to start. She had always wanted to hike in the Smoky Mountains, and that's how she found me. She signed up for a retreat and started showing up for our Retreat Training calls. The retreat training focuses on starting people where they at, and she was at a beginner level. No problem. Everyone is a beginner at some time! But she was fighting the feeling that time was running out, and she had to GET GOING right now, full out. Her body wasn't ready for what she was trying to do, and things started hurting. She'd had aches and pains from not moving in the past, but this was different. Suddenly she could tie her pain to something she was doing, and it wasn't pretty. With every call, she had a new pain and a new reason why she couldn't continue her training.

As we conversed, it became strikingly evident that at the core of her struggles lay a deep sense of inadequacy and a complete absence of joy. It didn't matter what activity she engaged in; the feeling persisted. The notion of embracing a beginner's mind felt like a failure to her. She believed there was no time to fiddlefart in the process of learning and attempting new things, which only resulted in recurring injuries and persistent discomfort.

Eventually, we hit on a plan that worked for her. Her favorite thing to do was dance, so we found a dance workout that checked a lot of the boxes for her retreat training, and she agreed to start doing her mobility every day. It sounded lame (her words, not mine), but once her body got used to moving, she was able to switch it up, try new things, and rock that retreat! A beginner's mind allows you to go slow, be kind to yourself and be curious.

Sometimes, the action steps we need to take to get to the end result aren't as fun or exciting as the actual end result. This is an "in-the-moment" tool that is one of the most important ones in your toolbox. Think of it this way, when a child is learning to ride a bike, there is usually some, or a lot, of pain along the way. Crashes, bandaids, feelings of inadequacy, all the feels. But, there are wins, triumphant moments, and eventually, the feeling that only a ride through the neighborhood on a summer evening with your best friends can bring. A beginner's mind can bring some amazing blessings into our lives.

Grab your Freedom Journal now, and carry out this short exercise. In our next chapter, we'll touch on the other three fitness pillars, fuel, sleep, and less stress! No fitness plan is complete without considering how these areas impact your health and energy.

KEY TAKEAWAYS, ACTIONS, AND JOURNAL PROMPTS

Before you move on to the next chapter, grab your freedom journal and do two things:

1. Write down three tools in your toolbox that you are willing to try next time you feel like you have zero motivation.

_____

_____

_____

Make a list of 3-5 (or more) things you'd like to try. Activities you are willing to have a beginner's mind around. Sprinkle them over the next couple of months. This is all about fun, freedom, and embracing joy. It has ZERO to do with the scale, the worry or anything else that might be cluttering your mind a bit. It's time to choose fun!

_____

_____

_____

CHAPTER 12
THE FOUR FITNESS PILLARS

Sometimes we 'hope' that if we're following our fitness plan to a T, we can slip up in other areas, eat whatever we want, steal from our sleep to create time for something else, and burn the candle at both ends to get it all done.

It doesn't work that way. Especially as the years add up.

I would be remiss to not mention the other fitness pillars (outside of movement). These work together to make us our healthiest possible selves; movement, fuel, restorative sleep, and less stress. Much like the four legs of a table, they are integral to supporting your fitness journey. Without some focus on each of them - everything eventually topples. I'm not into hard and fast rules - but the longer I have worked with my clients and focused on my own health, the more clear it has become to me that without these four essentials, it is almost impossible to build a strong fitness foundation.

What I've included in this chapter are some simple suggestions to consider. Don't do everything at once, but just become aware of the pillars and add them in as you have the bandwidth. Small changes can make big differences.

If you're eating whatever you want or indulging in excessive sugar while hoping that your workouts will offset poor nutrition, you may have found that this no longer works! Or, maybe sleep is your bailiwick, and you try and convince yourself that you're a unicorn, one of those people who can get by on 4-5 hours of sleep. But, time and time again, studies show that the majority of people need 7-9 hours of sleep to maintain physical, neurological, and emotional health. Yes, it might feel almost impossible to find this much time to sleep, but I've got you covered with suggestions in this chapter.

Let's dive into these pillars and how to make them work for you!

The Right Fuel to Feed Your Body

I am not a nutritionist, and I'll be the first to say I have no letters behind my name or medical training, but I know for a fact that what goes in our bodies either takes care of us or depletes us. We have to fuel our bodies with the right food/fuel at the right time.

I'm not talking about a diet. Diets typically focus on taking things away - I prefer to add things in. Think good, healthy, whole food. Food that gives your body the fuel it needs to do what you want it to do. Vegetables, fruits, grains, clean proteins, whole grains, all the goodness!

Everyone is different, and you need to find a way of eating that works for you, one that gives your body what it needs and gets it where it wants to go. My general rule of thumb has evolved and changed over the years. At one time, I could literally exercise off the extra calories I consumed with longer bouts of cardio. Now, longer bouts of cardio contribute to muscle loss and fat gain, so I somewhat limit my long cardio and my calories!

Our bodies need the right fuel to do everything we want to be able to do. As we accumulate more life experiences, our bodies undergo natural wear and tear and changes. Because of this, food as fuel becomes more important than ever. We need to be able to wring every single bit of nutrition from our fuel.

There are so many excellent books on sources for optimal nutrition. A couple of my current faves are *The Blue Zones Solution* by Dan Buettner and *Food, What the Heck Should I Eat* by Dr. Mark Hyman are good places to start. Food is personal, and ultimately, our choices and food and nutrition relationship are different for each of us.

My best suggestion is to eat the healthiest, most earth-friendly foods you can. Opt for organic when possible, the least amount of processed foods you can find, read labels and avoid added sugar. You will probably find that you need to increase your protein input. As we pass fifty, our desire for protein begins to wane as our need for protein increases. To reach protein levels that support muscle, you will most likely find that you need a protein supplement. The science of supplements is evolving on a daily basis. I've added my favorites to the book bonus section for easy access and discounts. Find what works for you, make sure you eat healthy and enjoyable food, track what you eat, and make small adjustments as you go.

Restorative Sleep

A good night's sleep is crucial for restoring our bodies and minds, allowing us to tackle a new day refreshed. There are some people who can get by with minimal sleep, but the reality is that almost all of us need a good strong seven-plus hours of sleep. A good night's sleep does so much. It regulates our emotions. It restores our bodies. It restores our brains. I am such a huge proponent of a good night's sleep that if I have to choose between a good night's sleep or getting up early for a workout, sleep will win out almost every single time. Not only will a good night's sleep allow you to tackle a new day rested and refreshed, but it cuts down on cravings and urges. Empty carbs, sugar, and too much caffeine are all triggered by a lack of sleep. Sleep is a bodybuilder.

Along with everything else, getting a good night's sleep can play a significant role in weight loss efforts. Studies have found that inadequate sleep can interfere with hormones that regulate hunger and appetite, leading to increased cravings for high-calorie and high-carbohydrate foods.[1] Furthermore, sleep deprivation has been linked to elevated levels of cortisol, a hormone that promotes fat storage, making weight loss more challenging.[2]

In contrast, getting sufficient sleep has been linked to a healthier weight status. A research study concluded that individuals who received an adequate amount of sleep (between seven and nine hours per night) were more successful in achieving weight loss and maintaining it compared to those who were sleep deprived.[3] Here are a few key tips for optimal sleep:

- *Avoid using your bed for activities other than sleep and sex:* Using your bed for activities like work or watching TV can create a mental association between bed and wakefulness, making it harder to fall asleep.

- *Establish a regular sleep schedule:* Try to go to bed and wake up at the same time every day, even on weekends.

- *Create a relaxing bedtime routine:* Engage in relaxing activities like reading, taking a warm bath, or practicing meditation to help prepare your body for sleep. Stop screen time two hours prior to bedtime and remove your phone from the bedroom if possible. If not possible, place it out of sight with all notifications and sounds turned off.

- *Ensure your sleeping environment is conducive to sleep:* Keep your bedroom cool, dark, and quiet to promote restful sleep. Consider a Chili Pad- Sleep if you cannot keep your room cool enough or have a partner who objects to sleeping cold.me, it's one of my favorite devices I own!

- *Limit caffeine, sugar, and alcohol.* They are sleep disruptors, especially in the hours leading up to bedtime.

- *Avoid eating heavy meals close to bedtime:* Digestion can interfere with sleep, so it's best to eat lighter meals earlier in the evening.

- *Get regular exercise:* Regular exercise can improve sleep quality, but avoiding vigorous exercise close to bedtime is important.

- *Limit exposure to screens before bedtime:* The blue light emitted by electronic screens can disrupt the sleep-wake cycle, so it's best to avoid screens for at least an hour before bedtime.

- *Manage stress:* Stress and anxiety can interfere with sleep, so it's important to find healthy ways to manage stress, such as practicing relaxation techniques or seeking professional help if needed.

- *Calm your mind before bed:* If you have a busy mind that seems to turn on as you turn off the lights, keep a journal next to your bed and do a quick brain dump of any racing around in your mind. Calming worry will help you sleep!

- *Don't panic if you wake up in the middle of the night:* Relax, count sheep, read a book using a redlight headlamp (avoid blue light that can disturb your circadian rhythm)

- *Track your sleep:* Use a sleep-tracking device like Oura Ring, but only if you will find the data interesting and not disturbing!

- *Consider sleep-promoting supplements or teas:* Certain supplements or teas, such as melatonin or chamomile, may help promote sleep, but it's important to consult with a healthcare provider before trying any new supplements.

Incorporating these tips into your daily routine can help improve sleep quality and promote overall physical and mental well-being. It's important to prioritize getting adequate sleep for optimal health and functioning.

Fit is Freedom Friend - Lynn

Lynn joined our 12-week accelerator program, determined to lose weight and gain muscle. With an impending surgery on the horizon, she wanted to be in the best possible shape she could be. She was on fire. Every week I could see her results in our online portal. The weight was coming off, and so were the inches. Her food choices were changing, and she was tracking everything she ate and all of her workouts. I was super impressed. When her weight started to plateau, we got on a call.

I asked her what she wanted to focus on, assuming we'd discuss ways to get out of a plateau, but she completely surprised me. *"My biggest issue right now is my sleep. I just naturally thought when I had less stress in my life, my sleep would improve, but it hasn't. I'm getting worried!"*

We went over her sleep habits, and she was doing a lot of things right. I made a few suggestions, like limiting social scrolling in bed, using a red light headlamp to read before sleeping, and how to fall back asleep when she woke up in the middle of the night. That's when we hit the problem.

"I don't go back to sleep."

"Excuse me?" I said. *"If you wake up at 3:00 to go pee, you just get up then?"*

"Yep, I figure I'm not going to fall back to sleep, so I just get up."

We made a plan. One that I know she did not completely buy into, but she gave it a try. Instead of worrying about the fact she was awake at 3AM and might as well get up, we came up with several options for what she could do. She could count sheep :), she could read with a redlight headlamp, and she could turn on a meditation. The one thing she couldn't do was get up before 6AM. What we really did was give her permission to go back to sleep. If it took a while to fall asleep, she might sleep in a little, but sleep was the focus. The crazy thing? Within a month, she slept better than ever and still is. She now loves her sleep!

Sleep restores us, our bodies, our brains, and our emotions.

Stress…Less

We simply must learn to stress… less. Stress negatively affects so many body systems, from hormones to digestion, cardiovascular and mental health, and sleep. One result of excess stress is that as our cortisol increases, so does our weight - especially around the belly![4] When we are stressed, we get triggered easier, and from there, it's a toxic cascading domino effect. Our bad habits come rushing to the forefront. Fortunately, there are some ways to deal with stress that I will share next. Of course, they are not as good as fixing the root cause of stress, which you should try doing, but these simple methods can make a visible difference.

Awareness

When we stop and become aware that we are feeling or reacting in a stressful manner, we have the option to become still. Stillness removes stress. You can stop and simply do a quick round of mindful box breathing; breathe in for the count of four, hold for the count of four, release for the count of four, and hold for the count of four. Make up your own breathing pattern, whatever works for you. Awareness and breathing are simple patterns to interrupt a stressful situation.

Other ways of managing stress healthfully are to journal, sing, dance, move, go outdoors, meditate, or grab your freedom journal and list three to five things you are grateful for and truly feel your gratitude. There's no room for stress and gratitude at the same time. If you are in an unmanageable situation, find support outside of your typical channels - break the cycle.

Daily Movement

This book is about fitness, after all! You have to move every day. I'm not talking about daily gym grinds or exercise classes that leave you exhausted, just movement. On days that your fitness plan doesn't call for a workout or a strenuous cardio session, enjoy a gentle walk outside, take the stairs instead of the elevator, do some yin yoga before bed, anything that gets the blood flowing and connects you to your body.

Revisiting your MDM (minimum daily movement)

If you skipped your MDM while building your custom plan, you're not alone. Most of my clients initially believe they don't need a minimum daily movement, they have a plan, and they're going to follow it! Which is fantastic; I applaud, and I know that life happens. When we get thrown off our usual schedule, we need a simple movement plan to fall back on. For me, it's very simple. If I'm experiencing a day where it looks like my schedule is going to be thrown off, I opt for either a little mobility (5 - 10 minutes tops) and a walk or maybe a little mobility and a couple of nitros. I don't look at this as part of my fitness plan, I look at it as a simple way to keep the systems in my body working well.

As I mentioned at the beginning of this chapter, just start considering these pillars. Don't do everything at once but start small and make changes as you have time. Small changes always add up to big results. There's another piece to this fitness journey that no one ever wants to acknowledge, but knowledge is power, and in the next chapter, we're going to touch on what happens when you experience an injury or physical setback.

CHAPTER 13
SOMETIMES IT MIGHT HURT

"I'm not saying this to worry you but to make you aware. Sometimes you might hurt. It could simply be the pain of lactic acid as you gain muscle, a strain, or it might even be recovering from a surgery. Aches and pains do happen, it's how we handle it that is going to make the difference in your life." Kelly

Leigh was new to the active lifestyle. Years of overwork, too much stress, and a little too many nights partying had taken a toll. She came to me when she was 59 and had been told by her doctor she was prediabetic and her blood pressure was too high. Her doctor had suggested she start on an exercise plan, and she had no idea of what to do or how to do it. Since she lived in the center of Los Angeles, I knew her options of what she had available were almost unlimited.

After going over her history of aches and pains, what she had tried (not much, water aerobics a few years back), and what she liked to do (dance and walk), I suggested she start out with a Yin Yoga class twice weekly and a beginner's pilates class twice weekly, plus a couple of walks. I wanted her to start slow, and she could build up as she and her body got used to the movement. Two days after our first call, she texted me in a panic. *"Something is wrong with my back, I've hurt myself."*

I was worried and asked her to get on a conference call with me ASAP. We jumped on a call, and she started by touching her lats and her triceps, saying, *"It hurts when I raise my arms or reach forward."* Hmmm, it looked like she was experiencing a little lactic acid buildup for possibly the first time in her life. To be 100% careful, I asked her to make an appointment with a physical therapist and suggested a soak in a warm bath, tossing in some Epson salts as a bonus. A day later, she texted me to let me know she wasn't hurting anymore. Most likely lactic acid, but I still asked her to go to PT.

A week later, I got another frantic text, *"I've hurt my knees."* I texted back, *"Both of them? Did you fall?"*

"No, I went on a longer walk than normal, and now they hurt, I don't know what to do."

She was in a panic state, so we jumped on another conference call, and I asked her what was different on this walk other than going further than usual. On our group call that week, one of the ladies had talked about doing stairs every week. She was in great shape and was training for a big hiking adventure. Leigh had decided to give the stairs in her parking garage a go and had made it up and then back down eight flights.

I complimented her, suggested she make another PT appointment, and suggested a little ice and some mobility (which she hadn't done before her walk). She was fine the next day, but I insisted on a visit to the PT for a light massage.

When the third frantic text came just a few weeks later, I called her directly to see what happened. As she explained another (potentially) use issue, I said, *"Leigh, sometimes it's going to hurt. Your choice is to decide if it's going to hurt from you learning to move and use your body or if it's going to hurt from unuse. When muscles and joints start aching from not being used, heart issues arise, or predi-*

abetes turns into diabetes." I wasn't trying to be harsh, but things can hurt when people begin an exercise program, especially when they've done zero to nothing in the past.

I've had my share of muscle aches, injuries, broken bones, and surgery followed by inactivity.

In fact... As I finish this book, it's been a strange couple of years for me. Two skin cancer surgeries followed by a broken arm took me out of most activities for almost six months last year. Then, I thought I would make up for lost time, and I pushed my weight training past what I should have (I knew better!!) and ended up with tendonitis in my elbow, and the only way it would get better was to slow down yet again. I wasn't going to mention these issues, but it seems dishonest not to share some of the trials I face too. What ended up being about eight months of limited movement took a toll on my body. But there are only two options. Give up or dig in.

As I went back and forth on this chapter, I decided it would be unfair not to share what I've learned over decades of being active and being sidelined at times. Life can be messy, unexpected aches and injuries do happen. How you handle your body, setbacks, and your mindset makes all the difference. Injuries are as much a mental game as a physical recovery!

Note: Contact your medical specialist when you experience injury, pain, or ongoing issues. The following ideas are suggestions only. Please use your best judgment!

Mind Your Mind

Your mind is your best friend and sometimes your worst enemy, the source of your biggest blocks. The more you move, the more your brain releases dopamine. It's a good addiction. A body in motion wants to stay in motion. You get used to the good feelings that movement produces. When you are suddenly sidelined from whatever might have happened, it doesn't take long before the lack of movement translates into increased stress, mood swings, and less sleep. You have goals, a workout schedule, and a routine, and then suddenly, you can't do them. You feel like you're crawling out of your skin and don't know what to do. You're not wacky. You're experiencing what happens when you suddenly stop moving!

Many years ago, a friend called early one Saturday morning. It was an unusual time for us to chat, so I immediately picked up, thinking she needed me to come get her from the side of the road somewhere, she was in training for a triathlon, and maybe her bike broke down.

Nope, it wasn't her bike…all I had to say was, *"How are you?"* and the tears started rolling. She could barely catch her breath as she started telling me about an unexpected surgery she had about six weeks before (I had no idea, but in hindsight, she had been strangely silent). As she sobbed into the phone, I finally got her to take a breath and stop so I could ask her, *"Have you been able to do anything, or are you bedridden?"*

"Bedridden," she sobbed.

Between her tears, I started explaining what was going on in her brain. She wasn't losing it like she thought, she was literally having exercise withdrawal. It happens, and it's all about how you work with it. If you find yourself in this situation, ask yourself: how can I make this work for me?

When I was sidelined from my leg surgery, I knew I'd be off my leg for eight weeks. That's a long time, and I had to make it work for myself, or I'd be sobbing into the phone too! Instead of getting to go hiking or biking those weekends, I recorded podcasts and worked. I knew that if I did some extra work while my leg was out of commission, I could take time off when my leg was healed and hit the trails. I made it work.

Another way to look at an injury is as if it were a gift. If this injury was a gift, what would it be? For me, I always go back to the morning I woke up in so much pain that I couldn't move. No doubt, I spent a couple of days wallowing and feeling like a victim. Worrying, will I never be able to move again? Is this my new normal? I definitely let my inner drama queen take center stage and go to my head. After those first couple of days, I was able to reign it in and think, what if this was a gift? What would that gift be for me?

The gift my injury brought was, I realized, time to change my business. I would have never had the time to grow and make changes in my business without this injury. All my wailing and laying on my back in pain drove me to this driving desire to help all the women that come to me to feel better, to have more fitness, more consistency, and more freedom. That was my gift. What would that gift be for you? It could simply be getting some time to kick back and rest or do a jigsaw puzzle. Whatever the gift may be for you, try to think about it like that.

Move Your Attention

Once you find the gift in your injury, the next piece is moving your attention. It's easy to focus on what's not working, but that can lead to a downward spiral. Instead, move your attention to something different. It could be relaxation and a jigsaw puzzle or taking a class you've wanted to take but haven't found the time. Catch up with friends. Take time to declutter. If you have things you need to clean up or straighten out, now is the time.

It's also a great time to deal with your gear. By gear, I'm talking about anything you need to do the things you love. When I was injured, I took the time to really look at all my hiking gear, specifically my hiking clothes. I found that they were all pretty old – I'm talking 10+ years old – and looking rough. I finally had that time to go through my hiking gear and see what I needed to replace. Once I was healed and able to get out and play, all my gear was ready to go.

When you can't do the things you want to do, find the things that you need to do. The bottom line is, don't be a victim. It is so easy to feel sorry for ourselves when we can't do what we want to do. There is a time for wallowing because everyone needs to take a moment to get those feelings out. But once the wallow is over, move your attention and get back to what needs to be done.

Pivot, When Possible

I like to call this "fitness flipping." Ask yourself, "What can I do given the situation I am in right now?" Let's say the doctor told you not to do anything from the waist down. Focus on the waist up! Maybe it's time to get serious about upper body strength or core workouts. What can you do, try, or double down on? I spent more time on my stationary bike and hiking when I had tennis elbow. When my client broke her ankle, she bought a waterproof cast cover and spent more time kayaking. If you love running, but the concrete is causing issues, try hiking on trails. It's all about thinking outside of the box and looking for options!

Get Creative

Try something new. You might try something new for healing. Over the years, I have tried all kinds of options. I've tried acupuncture, body and mind integration, nutrition, trigger balls, supplements, red light therapy, and more. They all helped me in some way. Trying new healing modalities opens your mind to new possibilities.

I was leading a surfing trip in Costa Rica a few years ago. I'm not a surfer. I want to be, but quite frankly, I suck at it. About six weeks before the trip, I fell off a horse and broke my arm. As I was getting a cast on my arm, I was in a panic, "I need to heal ASAP!" I had no time to waste, I was going on a trip in six weeks. Not just any old trip, a surfing trip!

No way I was staying home. I asked the doctor about what supplements he suggested I take to heal quicker. He looked at me like I was crazy and just said, *"Yep, try all the supplements you want…but it's still going to take eight weeks to heal."* Well, that's fair, but I was still going to try everything. I told him I would be back in four weeks to see how things were healing. He looked at me and just nodded.

I went back in five weeks – my trip a week away – and I was sure my arm was ready. Once the doctor took the cast off, the pain immediately returned. It was not healed. The doctor was a great guy and started getting into the spirit of the surfing trip when he said, *"I have an idea for you. What if this next cast stops below your elbow? Then you can bend your elbow and try doing whatever you think you can do."* The first cast had gone from my wrist to my shoulder, so my entire arm was immobilized. Having a shorter cast would absolutely give my arm more freedom! A shorter cast was added, and I bought a waterproof cast cover. Off I went on that surfing trip. I wasn't the surfer I dreamed of being, but I could paddle and get up on the waves, that was good enough for me! And I took my doctor a signed photo of me surfing as a joke when I returned to have the cast removed for good.

He just shook his head ●.

If you need to get creative, what can you do? How can you think outside the box? Even if your injury is not a broken bone but an issue with joints or ligaments, there are things you can do to heal. Maybe use a massage gun, trigger balls, or even mobility exercises. How can you help your body start healing? Sleep is another method of healing that may be overlooked. The more deep sleep we get, the better we heal. You can also try visualizing or meditation as a way to heal (or at least calm your mind). These are just some ways you can get creative and think outside the box for healing.

Case Study/Storytime

I'm a big fan of using trigger balls when body parts hurt. If you haven't heard of or used a trigger ball before, it is simply a hard ball that you press into a trigger point or muscle to relieve pain and tension.

One day I went hiking with a client, it was a longer hike than I had planned and ended up being about three hours. When we returned, my client was tired and went home to nap. A couple of hours later, she texted me, *"You broke me,"* and I just smiled and replied, *"What do you mean I broke you?"*

She said, *"My feet hurt so bad. I can't walk."* I said, *"Okay. Let's do something about it. I want you to use your trigger balls on your feet."*

In disbelief, she said, *"I can't do that. My feet are bruised beyond belief. I am in pain."*

I told her, *"I'm betting that with the good boots you had on your feet, they aren't bruised beyond belief. Maybe the muscles are a little bit irritated, and the trigger ball might help."* So she trusted me, used her trigger ball, and then gave her feet some rest, and sure enough, they were fine later that day. The moral of the story is to be willing to do things and be creative.

Avoid Injuries

The next piece is simply avoiding injuries. We can all do it to a large degree. One of the first places I see people getting injured is they start out too fast, too hard, or do too much. Another key is knowing the difference between muscle soreness and an injury. You can work through muscle soreness and rest an injury. Of course, I'm not a doctor, but over time, I see the women I work with learning their bodies and when to push and when to slow down!

If you're an athlete, you know that there is even a difference between lactic acid building up in your muscles and something that's not right. So slow down and don't overdo it.

Know the difference. Even if you work with a trainer or take a class led by a trainer, trust yourself. I've seen injuries from over-exuberant trainers who push people harder than they should be pushed. Care for your joints and start slow.

I've been in a Pilates class where the instructor told me I was doing it wrong and needed to do it this way. I kindly told her, *"Thank you for the input, but my shoulder can't handle that, and I need to do it my way. If I try to do it the way you want me to, there is going to be an issue."* She backed off, and I backed off on doing something that would hurt me. So trust yourself and know your body. Be willing to say 'no' when you think someone is giving you bad advice. Do not let your ego worry about what someone else will think. If you really believe it's bad for your body, your joints, or where you are physically in the moment, just say, "Thank you but no thanks!"

Another way to avoid injuries is by practicing mobility and balance. These are movements that are going to keep us going for a long time. Work on mobility and balance today, and tomorrow will take care of the rest!

The last piece for avoiding injury is simply moving. Movement is what our body needs. Start small with easy, gentle movement. Through movement, your body and brain heal. It may take time, but remember, our bodies are resilient. Take care of yourself today, and you'll have so many more good days to enjoy.

Remember to mind your mind, shift your attention, pivot when needed, get creative, and avoid injuries whenever possible. If you're sidelined, it won't be for long because once you're an athlete at heart, you're an athlete for life.

Congratulations on getting here! In the next chapter, you'll find a road map that lays out the steps we have gone through. Keep this list as a quick-check guide for any time you need a reminder or a boost.

CHAPTER 14

YOUR ROAD MAP TO FITNESS FREEDOM

Let's recap what we learned in the book and get ready for a fit and free future. You'll also find a printable copy of this Fitness Road Map in your Freedom Journal. Use this to keep yourself on track and back on track anytime you need a little insight.

We started with…

Step 1. *Start with your North Star.* What will fit, fun and free mean for you? More life in your life? More energy and confidence? More quality time with those you love? Write it out! Post it on your wall if you need to.

Step 2. *You are the priority.* When my clients say, *"I need to make myself the priority,"* it is almost always a sotto voce remark the first few times. It feels wrong to put ourselves first. You must realize that when you find time for your fitness and well-being, you're giving those you love a future filled with the love only you can give them. You are creating years of life brimming with health and happiness. There's nothing in this world that is a more caring gift for those you love.

Step 3. *Schedule your weekly workouts.* Every week. Your schedule should include cardio, strength, mobility/stretching, and rest days. Have an MDM (minimum daily movement) already created so those days that life gets messy, you're still setting yourself up for a better day tomorrow.

Step 4. *Practice awareness.* What is stopping you? If it's no time, adjust your schedule. If it's no desire, go back to your North Star. If it's an injury or pain, do everything in your power to get well. Do what you need to do to get moving again and feel great.

Step 5. *Throw everything you can at this.* What you do today impacts the rest of your life. Positively or negatively. Use accountability. Community. Fitness besties. Have something to look forward to. Use layered accountability. Find a community, a coach, or an app, create your weekly workout schedule, and stay focused on your why. Take advantage of my complimentary reader discovery call and book a quick chat HERE: www.fitisfredom.com/call. Use everything you have and have learned. In the end, the responsibility for how you feel for the rest of your life comes back to you. When you're 100% committed, it works. When you're 99% committed… there's always a way out.

Step 6. *Pay attention when the consistency killers show up.* Perfection, roadblocks, going past your tipping point, being overbooked, overwhelmed, and your personal Kryptonite can all pose massive hurdles to your growth. Striving for perfection doesn't work; 80% is good enough. Worrying that things aren't happening fast enough will slow you down. Ruminating about the past accomplishes nothing. Stay in the moment and keep moving forward. Anticipate roadblocks and be aware of when you might be overbooking yourself. Use your MDM and look for easy ways to make your schedule work. Slowing down on working out for a week or two is fine; just don't stop.

Step 7. *Motivation slipping? A body in motion stays in motion!* Movement creates motivation, not the other way around. Get moving, and do everything you now know how to do to get back on track. Use this book, my podcast, other fitness podcasts and books, meditation, and journaling. Keep your freedom journal by your side. Keep a toolbox of options. Don't sweat if your schedule slips for one or two days; restart. If a week slips by without working out, dig in and go back through steps 1-7.

And finally, we covered how to …

Step 8. *Get ready for more!* What is next? Make plans, have things to look forward to, and live life fully and have fun. Focus on your North Star and remember to ask yourself, what does living a life of Fun, Fitness, and Freedom look and feel like for me?

And then BEGIN!

Here's What's Next

As our journey together comes to a close, I'm ecstatic that your fitness journey is just beginning. You now know the path to Fitness Freedom is seldom a straight line, but you have everything you need to succeed. There may be side trips and missteps, and you might occasionally find yourself starting over. I can't say this enough: It doesn't matter! You are never starting from the same place you started from originally. You'll always restart from a better foundation and a stronger, healthier body. There will be so many times when you realize how invincible you are, and I can't wait to meet along the way and maybe even share an adventure or two!

Here's to you for picking up this book and being willing to keep going, try harder, play bigger, and do everything you need to be the healthiest version of yourself possible. There is too much fun, love, and adventure to be had in this one precious life, not to give it our all.

You've got this!

I can't wait to share the view from the top of the mountain with you.

Hugs - Kelly

P.S. If you would like my help, I am here for you. It is absolutely possible for you to achieve everything you want on your own. And I know that having support can make this easier and faster. Like our Fit is Freedom Member Kay said: "I could have figured this out on my own, but the truth is I never did! At my age, I need to get going much sooner than I'd like to admit. This has worked for me better than I ever expected. Thank you!"

If you have questions, please get in touch with me at:

FitisFreedom.com/call

Don't forget to pick up all your bonuses at:

FitisFreedom.com/Bonuses

Ready to join me on a Retreat - awesome!

FitisFreedom.com/Retreat

BOOK BONUSES EMPOWER YOUR FITNESS JOURNEY

How to Get More Help:

I firmly believe in imperfect action AND having all the resources possible to move forward! In the spirit of "throwing everything at your fitness journey," I have curated a collection of free resources that will serve as your companion in this transformative endeavor. Consider these resources as a window into my work with my one-on-one clients—an expression of gratitude for being here and a hands-on approach to achieving tangible results.

To access these valuable tools, click on the links below, which will take you to a privately hosted portal designed exclusively for your convenience:

The Fitness Workout Builder

Embark on a guided quiz that will walk you through essential questions required to create your personalized workout plan. No worry about not being sure what steps to take, you'll have a custom-built plan ready for you in a matter of minutes! So, say goodbye to confusion and hello to a streamlined fitness journey. Access Link:

FitisFreedom.com/bonuses

PART 3

The Freedom Journal

Obtain your printable and/or editable copy of The Freedom Journal and join me on a transformative journaling experience. This invaluable resource will help you track your progress, reflect on your journey, and serve as a roadmap for your desired destination. From where you started to where you're headed, this journal will be your faithful companion every step of the way. Access link:

FitisFreedom.com/bonuses

1:1 Client Plan Creation Video Series

This very special video series has never been shared before. You'll feel like you're looking over my shoulder as I create fitness and adventure plans for my 1:1 clients. From Level One beginners to long-term enthusiasts, you'll gain insight into how I craft the exact results they yearn for—fun, fitness, and freedom. Prepare to be inspired and motivated. Access Link:

FitisFreedom.com/bonuses

Work With Me & My Team to Accelerate Your Results

I am here to guide you in living a life brimming with fun, freedom, and fitness. If the words within this book resonated with you and you seek my guidance in creating a fitness-focused life, I am ready to assist. I offer a diverse range of solutions tailored to your needs, including DIY digital courses, group coaching programs, personalized mentoring, and transformative retreats. Within this community, you will find a supportive network of like-minded women, fostering accountability and offering training options for every adventure you seek. Rest assured, there is a solution that aligns with your budget and will support and guide you towards a life where "Fit is Freedom."

So, don't wait, jump on a call. I am here to help.

FitisFreedom.com/call

Take a proactive step towards your fitness journey. Together, we can turn your aspirations into reality.

ABOUT KELLY

Kelly Howard is the Fitness Consistency Expert with a touch of Adventure! For over 25 years, she has helped busy women answer that all-important question: "What can I do NOW to fill the rest of my life with fun, fitness, and freedom?"

Kelly loves adding fun and adventure to life with outdoor activities like hiking, biking, backpacking, kayaking, and stand-up paddleboarding. She empowers women to adventure out of their comfort zones by trying outdoor experiences they have only dreamt of or possibly haven't experienced in a very long time.

Her Fit is Freedom podcast, coaching, online courses, and events have changed the lives of thousands of women. As a frequent guest on podcasts and television, she also created the FOX TV Outdoor Houston Adventure series. She currently calls Houston, Texas, home but can often be found kayaking rivers and traveling trails worldwide.

Website:

www.FitisFreedom.com

Facebook Group:

https://www.facebook.com/groups/kellyhoward

Podcast:

www.FitisFreedom.com/Podcast

Made in the USA
Monee, IL
01 August 2023